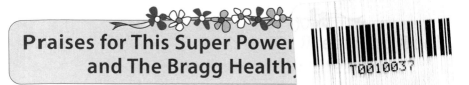

Praises for This Super Power [Breathing]
and The Bragg Health[...]

These are just a few of the thousands of testimonials we receive yearly, praising The Bragg Health Books for the super health and rejuvenation benefits they reap – physically, mentally and spiritually. We look forward to hearing your story, also!

Thanks to Paul Bragg and the Bragg Health Books, my years of asthma were cured in only one month with The *Bragg Breathing* and *Miracle of Fasting* Books and Bragg Healthy Lifestyle Living! – Paul Wenner, Gardenburger creator • *www.Gardenburger.com*

When I was a young gymnastics coach at Stanford University, Paul Bragg's words and example inspired me to live a healthy lifestyle. I was twenty-three then; now I am over sixty, and my health serves as a living testimonial to Bragg's health wisdom, carried on by his dedicated health crusading daughter, Patricia. Thank you! – Dan Millman, author *The Way of the Peaceful Warrior* • *www.peacefulwarrior.com*

Paul Bragg saved my life at age 15 when I attended the Bragg Health Crusade in Oakland, California. I thank Bragg Healthy Lifestyle for my long, healthy, active life spreading health and fitness. – Jack LaLanne, Bragg follower to 97 • *www.JackLaLanne.com*

As a youth I had a learning disability and was told I would never read, write or communicate normally. At 14 I dropped out of school and at 17 ended up in Hawaii surfing. My road to recovery led me to Paul Bragg who changed my life by giving me one simple affirmation to repeat: "I am a genius and I apply my wisdom." Paul Bragg inspired me to go back to school and get my education and from there miracles happened. I have authored 72 training programs and 40 books and love to crusade around the world thanks to Paul Bragg. – Dr. John Demartini, Dynamic Crusader, Star in *The Secret* • *www.DrDemartini.com*

Bragg Super Power Breathing makes the weak strong and helps make athletes olympic winning champions! – Bob Anderson, famous stretching coach • *www.stretching.com*

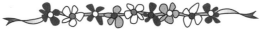

Just by paying attention to breathing, you can access new levels of health, energy and relaxation that will benefit every area of your life. – *Deepak Chopra, M.D.* • *www.chopra.com*

Improper breathing is a common cause of ill health. Changing your breathing patterns can affect and improve you mentally, emotionally and physically. – Andrew Weil, M.D.

Praises for This Super Power Breathing Book and The Bragg Healthy Lifestyle

In medical school I read Dr. Bragg's Health Books. They changed my way of thinking and the path of my life. I founded Omega Institute.
– Stephan Rechtschaffen, M.D.

Paul Bragg inspired me many years ago with the *Miracle of Fasting* and with his philosophy on health. His daughter Patricia is a testament to the ageless value of living the Bragg Healthy Lifestyle. – Jay Robb, author of *The Fruit Flush*

I have known Bragg Health Books for over 40 years. They are a blessing to me and my family and to all who read them to help make this a healthier world. – Pastor Mike MacIntosh, Horizon Christian Fellowship, San Diego, CA

Thanks to Bragg *Miracle of Fasting* and *Healthy Lifestyle* books, we're healthy, fit and singing better and staying younger than ever!
– The Beach Boys • *www.TheBeachBoys.com*

Your dad, Dr. Paul Bragg IS the FATHER of the natural health industry and the entire natural health movement. Everything that has been done in natural health and physical culture since has been based on the pioneering vision and principles articulated by Dr. Bragg. He gave us all our health direction!
– Dr. William Wong

I am following The Bragg Healthy Lifestyle which I heard of through a friend. Your books are motivators and have blessed my health and my life and are making the best perfect gifts for my family and friends. – Delphine, Singapore

Thanks to you and your wonderful father for your guidance and teaching over the years. What a great gift you and your father have provided for us all through your Bragg Health Books. Your Fasting and Vinegar books have improved my life immensely. I've lost 30 lbs. and feel years younger. At 67 youthful years, I give thanks for the great benefits of health I enjoy because of the work you and your father have so generously dedicated your lives too!!
Wishing you every blessing under the Sun.
– Captain Wes Herman (retired) Santa Barbara County Fire Dept.

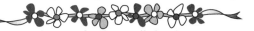

A laugh is just like sunshine, it freshens all the day. – Heart Warmers

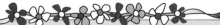

Praises for This Super Power Breathing Book and The Bragg Healthy Lifestyle

How I beat cancer, obesity, diabetes, strep and three herniated disks and excruciating pain? The answer was changing to the Bragg's Healthy Lifestyle and doing Super Power Breathing Exercises. It changed and saved my life! I had full recovery and I also lost 70 lbs. I received a new life and that is just the beginning because my manhood returned that was lost to diabetes – now that's exciting! On my trip to Honolulu, I visited the famous free Bragg Exercise Class at Waikiki Beach. I became so regenerated with a wonderful new viewpoint towards living the Bragg Healthy Lifestyle that I now live in Hawaii. I'm invigorated with new energy for life and living! My new purpose for living is to help others reclaim their health rights! I want the world to join The Bragg Health Crusade. I am deeply thankful to Paul and Patricia for my new healthy life!
– Len Schneider, Hawaii

Warm wishes all the way from Malaysia to express my sincere gratitude to both of you for sharing your precious health secrets of health and youthfulness with The Bragg Healthy Lifestyle Living!
– Marilyn Lim, Sarawak, Malaysia

I've experienced a beautiful, remarkable, spiritual and physical awakening since reading Bragg Books. I'll never be the same again.
– Sandy Tuttle, Painesville, Ohio

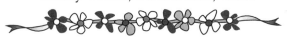

We get letters at our Santa Barbara Headquarters. We would love to hear from you on any blessings, healings and impact on your life you experienced after following The Bragg Healthy Lifestyle. It's all within your grasp to be in top health! By following this book, you can reap Super Health and a happy, long, vital life! It's never too late to begin – see pages 184-185, the study they did with people in their 80's and 90's and the amazing results that were obtained! You can receive miracles with nutrition, exercise and some fasting! Start now!

Daily our prayers & love go out to you, your heart, mind & soul.

Patricia and Paul C. Bragg

D

Miracles can happen every day through guidance and prayer! – Patricia Bragg

Patricia Bragg Books

Super Power
BREATHING

For Optimum Health & Healing

Empower Yourself • Energize Yourself • Relax Yourself

PAUL C. BRAGG, N.D., Ph.D.
LIFE EXTENSION SPECIALIST
and
PATRICIA BRAGG
HEALTH CRUSADER & LIFESTYLE EDUCATOR

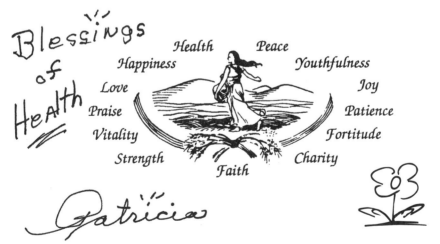

Blessings of Health

Health Peace
Happiness Youthfulness
Love Joy
Praise Patience
Vitality Fortitude
Strength Charity
Faith

Patricia

BECOME
A Health Crusader – for a 100% Healthy World for All!

www.PatriciaBraggBooks.com

Super Power
BREATHING

For Optimum Health & Healing

Empower Yourself • Energize Yourself • Relax Yourself

PAUL C. BRAGG, N.D., Ph.D.
LIFE EXTENSION SPECIALIST
and
PATRICIA BRAGG
HEALTH CRUSADER & LIFESTYLE EDUCATOR

Visit our website:
www.PatriciaBraggBooks.com

Twenty-sixth Edition MMXXI
ISBN: 978-0-87790-085-6

Library of Congress Cataloging-in-Publication Data on file with publisher

Published in the United States
HEALTH SCIENCE
7127 Hollister Avenue, Suite 25A, Box 249, Santa Barbara, CA 93117
Toll-Free: (833) 408-1122

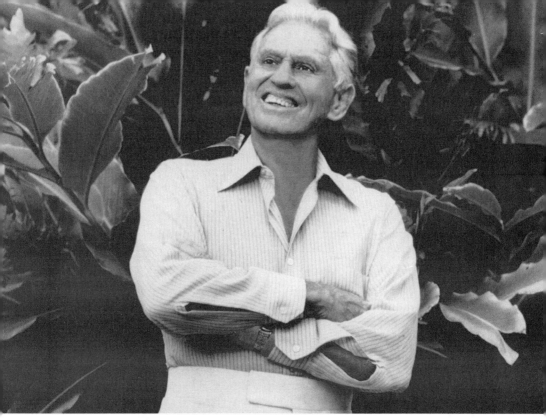

PAUL C. BRAGG, N.D., Ph.D.
World's Leading Healthy Lifestyle Authority

Paul C. Bragg's daughter Patricia and their wonderful, healthy members of the Bragg *Longer Life, Health and Happiness Club* exercised daily on the beautiful Fort DeRussy lawn, at famous Waikiki Beach in Honolulu, Hawaii. On Saturday there were often health lectures on how to live a long, healthy life! The group averaged 50 to 75 per day, depending on the season. From December to March it can go up to 125. Its dedicated leaders carried on the class for over 43 years. Thousands visited the club from around the world and carried the Bragg Health and Fitness Crusade to friends and relatives back home.

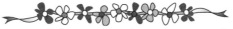

Your body is a non-stop living system, in constant motion 24 hours daily, cleaning, repairing, healing and growing. – Patricia Bragg

To maintain good health, normal weight and increase the good life of radiant health, joy and happiness, the body must be exercised properly (stretching, walking, jogging, biking, swimming, deep breathing, good posture) and nourished with healthy foods. – Paul C. Bragg, N.D., Ph.D.

iii

❁ Cautionary Note and Disclaimer ❁

The information provided here is for educational purposes only. Any decision on your part to read, listen and use this information is your personal choice. The information in this book is not meant to be used to diagnose, prescribe or treat any illness. Please discuss any changes you wish to make to your medical treatment with a qualified, licensed health care provider.

If you are taking medication to control your blood sugar or blood pressure, you may need to reduce the dosage if you significantly restrict your carbohydrate intake. This is best done under the care and supervision of an experienced and qualified licensed health care provider. Anyone who has any other serious illness such as cardiovascular disease, cancer, kidney or liver disease needs to exercise caution if making dietary changes. You should consult your physician for guidance. If you are pregnant or lactating, you should not overly restrict protein or fat intake. Also, young children and teens have much more demanding nutrient needs and should NOT have their protein or fat intake overly restricted.

The information presented in this book is in no way intended as medical advice or a substitute for medical counseling. It is intended only to provide the opinions and ideas of the authors. It is sold with the understanding that the authors are not engaged in rendering medical, health or any other kind of professional services in this book. The reader should consult his or her medical doctor, or any other competent professional, before adopting any of the suggestions in this book, or drawing inferences from it.

The authors disclaim any responsibility for any liability, loss or risk, personal or otherwise, which is incurred as a consequence, directly or indirectly, of the use and application of the contents of this book.

Please consult your physician before beginning this program, and use all of the information the authors suggest in conjunction with the guidance and care of your physician. Your physician should be aware of all medical conditions that you may have, as well as medications and supplements you are taking.

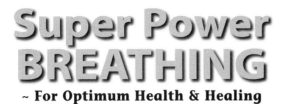

Super Power BREATHING

~ For Optimum Health & Healing

*To preserve health is a moral and religious duty, for health is the basis for all social virtues.
We can't be as useful when not well. – Dr. Samuel Johnson, Father of Dictionaries*

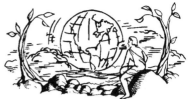

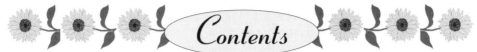

Contents

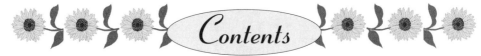

Contents

Contents

❧ ♥ ❧ Bragg Healthy Lifestyle Plan ❧ ♥ ❧

- *Read, plan, plot, and follow through for supreme health and longevity.*
- *Underline, highlight or dog-ear pages as you read important passages.*
- *Organizing your lifestyle helps you identify what's important in your life.*
- *Be faithful to your health goals everyday for a healthy, long, happy life.*
- *Where space allows we have included "words of wisdom" from great minds to motivate and inspire you! Please share your favorite sayings with us.*
- *Write us about your successes following The Bragg Healthy Lifestyle.*

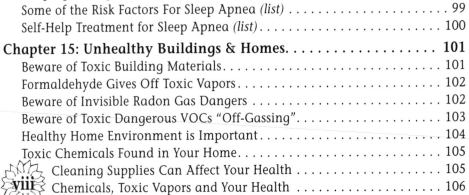

Contents

Contents

We all grow healthier in nature, gentle sunshine and love! – Patricia Bragg

Contents

No matter what your sense of direction, you'll never lose your way.
Your angel will always keep you on the right path. – Suzanne Siegel Zenkel

X

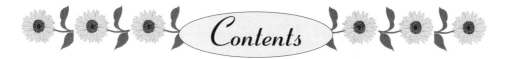

Contents

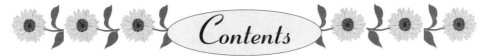

Contents

One of the most tragic things about human nature is that all of us tend to put off living. We are dreaming of some magical rose garden over the horizon – instead of enjoying the roses that are blooming outside our windows today.
– Dale Carnegie

The more natural food you eat, the more you'll enjoy radiant health and longevity and be able to promote the higher life of love and brotherhood.
– Patricia Bragg, Pioneer Health Crusader

When you live The Bragg Healthy Lifestyle you can help activate your own powerful internal defense arsenal and maintain it at top efficiency. But, bad or sloppy breathing habits make it harder for your body to fight off illness.

Chapter 1

Super Power Breathing For Super Energy

Do you know how to breathe?

The breath of life means exactly what it says: To breathe is to live; not to breathe is to die. A human can exist without food for weeks, go without water for days, but one can't exist for more than a few minutes without air!

This fact is so obvious and breathing is so automatic that most people take it for granted. *Yet, do you really know how to breathe?* Stop and think about it. Do you really know how your lungs function? Do you use these marvelous organs to their fullest? The way you use your lungs controls your life, your health, your looks, your energy, your resistance to disease – your very life span!

Super Power Breathing – The Path To High Vibration Energy Living

As health specialists with over a century of combined effort, we have developed techniques for measuring mental and physical energy in humans. Everyone lives at a certain rate of vibration. The human body is capable of reaching a high vibration energy level; unfortunately many never master what it takes to achieve this. Why? Because only a few know how to generate, utilize and replenish their full capacity of body and mind energy!

High vibration energy people are doers and achievers. They display seemingly inexhaustible vitality and stamina, creative power and/or athletic ability of the highest quality. They never seem to tire. They perform mental and physical tasks without strain or excessive emotion. To high vibration achievers, everything seems easy and effortless because they have more vital power!

Breathing is the most basic of bodily functions!

The Bragg Super Power Breathing habit of taking longer, slower, deeper breaths helps to produce more energy and a more vital, youthful, longer life for you!
– Paul C. Bragg, N.D., Ph.D., Life Extension Specialist, Originator of Health Stores

High Vibration Energy Produces Achievers

This natural energy produces contented people who see the humorous side of life: full of personal magnetism and enthusiasm. High vibration energy people are a joy to be with because they have happy dispositions. They are free from depressions and mental blocks, and are well-adjusted people who enjoy more fulfilling, healthy and happy lives. What is their secret? How do they live at a superior rate of high vibration energy? The answer is simple: such people consume large amounts of oxygen. They breathe deeply and fully, utilizing every square inch of their lung capacity. Ample oxygen combined with a healthy lifestyle does bring miracles.

The more oxygen you breathe into your lungs, the more energy you will have. This creates a higher rate of vibration. It is very much like a fire in an open burning fireplace, the more oxygen the fire gets, the brighter it will burn! The less oxygen it gets, the less heat and more unwanted smoke it generates – and soon the fire dies.

Most Live at Low to Medium Vibration

People who live at a low to medium rate of vibration attain limited levels of vitality, both mentally and physically. While they may have a capacity for work and play, they aren't capable of the sustained effort achieved by those who have high vibration energy. Low to medium vibration energy people easily tire and lack endurance, particularly when under stress. Exhaustion induced by tension and strain forces this type of person to stop, rest and sadly even give up.

People living even at a medium vibration rate simply don't get enough vital oxygen to give them that extra push to keep going under physical, mental or emotional pressures. Under extreme pressure they *run out of gas* and lack the high vibration energy that deep power breathing and healthy living provides to make this additional effort.

Our life-sustaining lungs fuel us with oxygen. We breathe in and out 22,000 times per day – processing about 300 cubic feet of air – just the amount needed to oxygenate 2,400 gallons of blood that is pumped through the heart daily.

Super Power Breathing Increases Energy

At age 16, my father, Paul C. Bragg, was diagnosed with a *hopeless* case of tuberculosis. Yet by age 18 he was cured and became a successful athlete. During those two years he was under the care of the great Swiss physician Dr. August Rollier. This wise doctor gave Dad a new lease on life with a regimen of all-natural healing methods. Using only pure distilled water, good nutrition, an apple cider vinegar drink, sunshine, fresh air, deep breathing and regular exercise, his body was able to cure itself with healthy natural living. After being healed, my father made a life-long pact with God to share his healthy lifestyle message with millions worldwide and he has!

Paul C. Bragg became a great-grandfather. He could out last most people half his age or less in any competition requiring energy and stamina. He easily typed for hours without mental or physical fatigue. He enjoyed hiking, jogging, biking, swimming, lifting weights, surfing, playing tennis and the challenge of climbing tall mountains around the world.

The Benefits of Effective Super Power Breathing

It is through breathing that we take in oxygen to fuel our minds and bodies. The more fuel we have, the better we function. The more effectively we breathe, the more effectively we live. Benefits of effective breathing include:

- increased oxygen intake
- balance of the emotions
- relief of stress
- relaxation of the body
- calming of the mind
- enhanced mental focus, clarity and creativity
- increased oxygenation of the blood, tissues, muscles and organs

Super Power Breathing can make your life-force stronger, calmer and smarter, which is wonderful when you stop and think about it – something so simple that can be so powerfully helpful and healthful to your total well-being!

Seek and find the best for your body, mind and soul. – Patricia Bragg

---

We can live for weeks without food, days without water, but only minutes without breathing. This tells us that breath and breathing is the element that's truly supplying our life-force on a minute by minute basis. We hope you are starting to see why breathing is so absolutely important to the body.

Count your blessings, name them one by one; count your many blessings, see what God hath done. – Johnson Oatman, Jr., songwriter
I give thanks for all the Miracle Blessings I receive daily. – Patricia Bragg

It's Never Too Late for You to Improve!

My father kept himself at a high rate of mental and physical vibration by supplying his body with the correct fuel: natural, healthy "live" foods and, above all, ample super power oxygen! He continually helped people in all walks of life – musicians, singers, writers, artists, doctors, lawyers, athletes, office workers and homemakers – to achieve a superior state of high vibration energy so they could enjoy Healthy Living. The basic source of super-oxygen-vibration is knowing how to deeply fill your lungs with oxygen. Everyone is born with this capacity, but unfortunately only a few retain this deep breathing habit naturally throughout life like athletes and singers do!

Whatever your age, it's never too late to learn how to increase your energy with the Bragg System of Super Power Breathing. After faithfully following the breathing exercises in this book, you too can soon learn how to fill your lungs with energy-producing, super power oxygen. You will enjoy the thrill of this great oxygen stimulation. It's far more potent than any toxic artificial stimulants such as alcohol, coffee, tea, cola and soft drinks and drugs. Plus oxygen has no side effects! In fact, deep oxygen stimulation can add up to a longer, healthier and happier lifetime.

The Miracle Surge of the Second Wind Helps Olympic Champions Win!

Why can't some get their *second wind*? It is because they are not using the full capacity of their miracle lungs for energy-producing oxygen. That is the big difference between the person who lives at the high vibration level and those who draw on only a medium rate of vibration. At a high rate of vibration, when you consume your full quota of oxygen, you are able to get your *second wind*. You feel stronger than when you started your effort. This miracle *second wind* is what makes high achievers, champion athletes, statesmen and women, writers, singers, actors, dancers and go-getters all equally high achievers.

Breathing is our connection to life, through the body & heart, leading us to a wholeness of being & giving us spirit for living life to its fullest. – S. Hainer, M.S.

When you learn to use the full capacity of your lungs through the Bragg System of Super Power Breathing, you will experience this wonderful stimulation of the *second wind.* Just when you think you have run out of energy, this sudden renewal of strength occurs! This is an experience truly difficult to describe. When you feel you cannot take another step, that your brain power is all gone, that your thinking is befuddled, then suddenly a great surge of energy courses through your entire body. You soon feel as fresh as, or even stronger than when you started! What a tremendous sensation! When you do this breathing correctly you experience this amazing *second wind!* **Many Olympic champions won their gold medals using Bob Anderson's wise help – the world's leading stretching coach teaches Bragg Super Power Breathing at seminars worldwide.**

Shallow Breathing Causes Premature Ageing

Regrettably, even the people who live at a medium rate of vibration are in the minority. In our modern world, most people are only half alive, existing merely at a very low rate of physical and mental vibration! Look around you – this includes people of all ages – from the early teens to the late 80's. Babies use their lungs as Mother Nature intended, but soon they acquire the unnatural, lazy, *civilized* habit of shallow breathing and begin to use only the top part of their lungs.

Shallow breathing starves the body of the oxygen it needs to be vitally alive! That's why there are so many people – from teenagers to oldsters – crowding doctors' offices, clinics, sanitariums, hospitals and convalescent homes. They drag themselves through life, seeking imaginary quick-fixes from artificial remedies in the form of laxatives, painkillers, tonics, sleeping pills and other popular, advertised over-the-counter drugs.

HEALTHY MIND HABIT: Wake up and say, "Today I am going to be happier, healthier and wiser in my daily living! I am the captain of my life and am going to steer it to living a 100% healthy lifestyle!" Fact is happy people look younger and have fewer health problems! – Patricia Bragg

---

The natural healing force within you is the greatest force in getting well. – Hippocrates, Father of Medicine, 400 B.C.

Oxygen-starved people are usually nervous and suffer from unnecessary worries as well as physical ills! Millions go to bed exhausted and wake up tired. They suffer from headaches, constipation, indigestion, muscular aches and pains, stiff joints, sore backs and feet, painful teeth and receding gums, poor eyesight and hearing, loss of memory, inflamed throats and respiratory ailments such as bronchitis, asthma, sinus infections and emphysema.

These health miseries and the loss of healthy bodily functions (which are often attributed to *ageing)* plague millions and sadly can take them to an early grave! They suffer and die needlessly – simply because they don't live a healthy lifestyle and most importantly, learn to breathe deeply and fully! It seems incredible, but with Super Power Breathing miracles happen! Prove it to yourself! **Life and health are priceless and should be treasured!**

Faith and Vision Create Miracles

Those happy, healthy, strong, vigorous people – who accomplish greatness – possess a deep spiritual philosophy. They believe that their lives are protected by a Power greater than their own. They believe there is a destiny that guides their lives. Nothing can stop them! Following the wise Laws of Mother Nature you can accomplish great miracles!

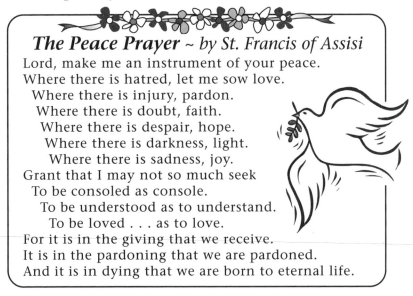

The Peace Prayer ~ by St. Francis of Assisi

Lord, make me an instrument of your peace.
Where there is hatred, let me sow love.
Where there is injury, pardon.
Where there is doubt, faith.
Where there is despair, hope.
Where there is darkness, light.
Where there is sadness, joy.
Grant that I may not so much seek
To be consoled as console.
To be understood as to understand.
To be loved . . . as to love.
For it is in the giving that we receive.
It is in the pardoning that we are pardoned.
And it is in dying that we are born to eternal life.

Chapter 2

Oxygen and Your Health
Oxygen Starvation

Suppose you are very hungry and sit down to enjoy a well-planned, nourishing meal . . . but as soon as you have eaten only a few bites of the food, someone snatches it away and tells you that you can't have any more! What would you think of the food-snatcher?

This is exactly what you do to yourself when you shallow breathe as most people do, using only 1/4 to 1/3 of your lung capacity! This starves your body more than if you were depriving it of food! You are slowly robbing your body of its most vital, invisible nourishment – oxygen!

Oxygen is essential to the ionization process, in which food molecules are broken down into nutrients suitable for the body's vital needs. Without sufficient oxygen your body cannot properly utilize the food you eat and drink, no matter how basically nourishing the food may be.

With an insufficient supply of life-giving oxygen, your blood slowly becomes saturated with poisonous carbon dioxide and other toxic wastes. It transports these toxins throughout your body (collecting more en-route), thereby suffocating your cells (also dulling brain cells), instead of rejuvenating them with sufficient life-giving oxygen!

Your brain, which requires three times more oxygen than the rest of your body, suffers first. Oxygen starvation is caused by shallow breathing, sedentary habits and the lack of exercise and fresh air! Educators who are alarmed about the decrease in the average student's IQ would do well to promote school physical education, exercise, sports and open windows! Tests and analyses are not brain food, but life-giving oxygen is!

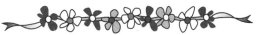

Breathing deeply, fully and completely energizes the body, calms the nerves, fills you with peace and helps keep you healthier and more youthful.
– Paul C. Bragg, N.D., Ph.D., Life Extension Pioneer

Rhythmic Breathing brings more air and oxygen into lungs and bloodstream.

Life-Giving Oxygen – Invisible Staff of Life

You can perform a simple demonstration by lighting two candles and placing them side by side, a few inches apart. Now partially cover one candle with a glass . . . watch how small and pale this flame becomes. If you cover the candle completely with the glass, the flame will go out in a few seconds. That is what happens in your body when you deprive it of life-giving oxygen.

The Heart and Blood Vessel Circulatory System

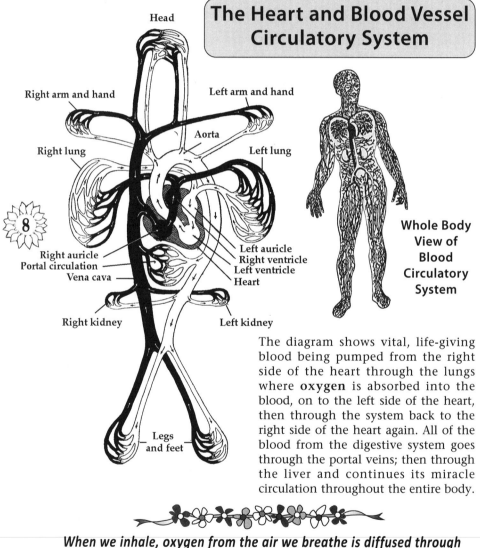

Head

Right arm and hand

Left arm and hand

Aorta

Right lung

Left lung

8

Left auricle
Right ventricle
Left ventricle
Heart

Right auricle
Portal circulation
Vena cava

Right kidney

Left kidney

Legs
and feet

Whole Body View of Blood Circulatory System

The diagram shows vital, life-giving blood being pumped from the right side of the heart through the lungs where **oxygen** is absorbed into the blood, on to the left side of the heart, then through the system back to the right side of the heart again. All of the blood from the digestive system goes through the portal veins; then through the liver and continues its miracle circulation throughout the entire body.

When we inhale, oxygen from the air we breathe is diffused through membranes and into red blood cells. The oxygen-rich blood then circulates throughout the body and finds tissues in need of oxygen.

Your heart and body take care of you and keep you alive – be good to them!

Oxygen Powers Your Miracle Human Machine

The human body is a miraculous intricate mechanism for the production of mental and physical energy. Oxygen, the invisible staff of life is this mechanism's power source. Your body begins to function with your first breath and continues until your last! How well it functions depends on your lifestyle and how well you supply it with oxygen!

As in any heat or combustion engine, **oxygen is essential to the production of energy in your body.** Every flame consists of the union of oxygen with other elements. The gasoline that fuels your car, the natural gas or coal in a heater or furnace and the wood in a fireplace or stove all contain latent energy. This energy cannot be released to produce the heat or power until its elements are broken down and united with life-giving oxygen!

This human body process is called metabolism. The food you eat contains latent energy, but it's of absolutely no use to you without oxygen. To determine the general health of our bodies, we can test the rate of our basal metabolism. This rate is determined in a laboratory by measuring the oxygen we use while our body is resting.

9

As long as you live, the body mechanism operates for you continuously. Even while asleep, your lungs, heart, kidneys, liver and other major organs, as well as circulatory and nervous systems, must continue to function 24/7! The amount of energy you need depends upon your mental and physical activities! **The release of energy you need depends upon your intake of oxygen and your general health.**

Oxygen is Carried by the Bloodstream

Every one of the over 30-40 trillion cells in your body demands a continuous flow of life-giving oxygen in order to stay alive, do its job and remain healthy! This oxygen supply is carried in your bloodstream by the red blood cells. There are millions of these red cells in every drop of your blood.

Increasing oxygen in your body helps to release toxins from the blood. Simplest form of increasing the body's oxygen is to do deep breathing exercises.
– Doris J. Rapp, M.D., author "32 Tips That Could Save Your Life"

Blood – Your Miracle River of Life!

The blood circulates in an average network of around 60,000 miles of blood vessels that reach every cell in the body, from those of the heart itself to the top of the scalp and to the tips of the fingers and toes. The average individual has about five to six quarts of blood circulating throughout their vast miracle body network at all times.

During rest or inactivity the blood makes on average one round trip per minute. During strenuous activity or exercise, however, it may make as many as eight or nine round trips per minute in order to supply the necessary fuel and oxygen for increased energy, and to help remove waste products and toxins from the body.

The blood vessels that carry blood from the heart are known as arteries. Those that return blood to the heart are veins. Both vary greatly in size and are organized just like streams, brooks and creeks flowing into a river, which joins a larger river.

The smallest blood vessels are called capillaries. They are so tiny that most are visible only under a microscope! Through these capillaries the last of the food and oxygen is given off and the return trip is made via the veins, which carry the oxygen-depleted blood and toxic wastes back to the heart for purification. En route to the heart, however, most of the water-soluble wastes are transferred to the kidneys for elimination through the urine. Poisonous carbon dioxide gas, a major residue of energizing oxidation, is brought back to the heart to be expelled through the lungs in breathing.

Super Power Breathing Detoxifies and Purifies Your Blood

The carbon dioxide collected from all parts of the body gives blood a blueish color when it is returned through the veins to the heart. There it enters the right auricle, the heart's upper chamber. After the auricle fills with blood, the valve into the right ventricle (lower chamber) opens, allowing the blood to pass into the ventricle. When the valve closes, the ventricle's strong muscles contract, sending blood to the lungs.

As blood travels through the capillary network in the lungs' air sacs, it discharges its load of carbon dioxide. It turns a healthy, bright red again as it absorbs the vital, life-giving oxygen before it immediately returns to the heart's left auricle. From there the blood flows into the left ventricle and by valve action is pumped vigorously into the body's largest artery, the aorta. Leaving the aorta, the blood then travels throughout the body via a vast arterial network – taking its life-giving oxygen and nutrients to every body cell to keep you healthy!

It is the shorter or *lesser* circulation – from the heart to the lungs and back – that is so vital to detoxifying and purifying the bloodstream! If the lungs are only partially filled with air, then only part of the bloodstream can be cleansed. The blood which passes through the capillaries of empty air sacs cannot get rid of its carbon dioxide waste and cannot pick up oxygen! So, instead of carrying a full quota of life-giving oxygen back to the cells of the body, the bloodstream returns with a mixture of fresh oxygen and a residue of toxic poisons. As this sluggish process continues, the proportion of carbon dioxide buildup increases, causing health problems!

11

How Oxygen Supports Body Detoxification

Health in the human body depends to a large degree on how efficiently nutrients can be absorbed and utilized at the cellular level, as well as how effectively the toxins and wastes can be removed! Cellular waste is removed from the body in several ways. Part of the waste is dissolved in water and transported to the kidneys and liver for filtration. It is then eliminated through the urine and bowels. Toxins are also excreted from the body through perspiration.

However, some of the most toxic poisons in the body can only be "burnt up" and neutralized through oxidation. This is the job of oxygen-rich red blood cells that circulate from the lungs and into the deeper organs and glands of the body.

Blood is the miracle river of life that flows through the human body. We cannot live without blood! The heart pumps blood to all our body's cells, supplying them with needed nutrition and oxygen.

Shallow Breathers Self-Poison Themselves

When you are a shallow breather, you don't change the air at the base of your lungs, where two-thirds of your lung capacity is located. When you return impure blood to your body, the ill effects are compounded because your blood cannot perform properly. It is difficult for blood that's loaded with poisonous wastes to transport the relatively small amount of oxygen which it absorbs; it's even harder for it to carry necessary nourishment from food. An inadequate oxygen supply impairs your body's ability to break down food into digestible elements. This slows all bodily function! This is why deep breathing is so vitally important for health!

With the wrong diet and shallow breathing, the organs of elimination are overworked and underfed! But accumulating wastes must go somewhere. Some are discharged into sweat glands. This toxic overload produces unpleasant body odors! Other toxic wastes end up deposited as heavy mucus into sinus cavities, lungs and bronchial tubes. Some line the passages of ears, eyes, nose and throat, as well as along the digestive tract. Deposits of hardened wastes in moveable joints can cause pressure on nerves, creating painful warning signals. **Pain is Mother Nature's flashing red warning signal that something is wrong in your body!** This pain warning should be respected with corrective measures taken right away – not repressed by painkilling drugs full of both known and unknown side-effects!

Shallow breathers actually poison themselves by robbing their bodies of sufficient oxygen! This is auto-intoxication (self-poisoning). They are slowly suffocating and dying in their own body wastes and poisons. **Pneumonia is a shocking example of this as the body and lungs fill up and the patient or victim drowns in their own toxins and mucus.**

Consider this: if someone tried to force you to kill yourself by taking shallow breaths, what would you do? You'd fight back! In defiance, you would breathe deeply, cleansing your blood and entire miracle body system to give your body more life, energy and super health!

Bragg Super Power Breathing helps make the weak strong and athletes champions.
– Bob Anderson, famous stretching coach to Olympic champions • stretching.com

Oxygen Deprived Cells Show Cancer Connection

Healthy cells in the body are aerobic, meaning they require adequate levels of oxygen for cellular respiration and growth! When cells are deprived of oxygen for any reason, decay sets in and the cells can mutate or die.

Dr. Otto Warburg, 1931 Nobel prize winner, discovered a close connection between oxygen and cancer. His studies showed that **the primary cause of cancer is directly related to oxygen-deprived cells!** In fact, he found that cancer cells are anaerobic and actually thrive in an oxygen-deficient environment.

Warburg also discovered that a slightly alkaline pH in the body meant higher levels of oxygen uptake. Now, having low blood oxygen levels is sadly a normal clinical finding for people with chronic diseases!

Increasing Your Body's Oxygen Naturally

Aerobic Exercise increases the level of oxygen in the body. Exercising such as brisk walking (page 178), swimming, cycling, dancing and mini-trampolining (rebounder) helps the heart and lungs to work more efficiently! When the lungs give the heart the oxygen it needs it doesn't have to overwork and is not as susceptible to heart attacks! Exercise for 30 minutes a day – 5 times a week is recommended.

Deep Breathing in a slow and relaxed way oxygenates and relaxes the body! Deep coordinated inhalation brings oxygen to the tissues, while deep exhalation helps move wastes from the body! Without proper breathing coordination, built-up tensions, etc. can cause breathing to become erratic and shallow. By consciously breathing deeper, you can bring benefits to both mind and body!

Fill Your Lungs with Super, Life-Giving Oxygen

Breath Expansion Test: Before beginning *Bragg Super Power Breathing Program*, perform this simple test. Exhale fully and measure deflated chest with a tape measure. Take a deep breath and measure again. After a month of practicing these exercises, take test again. You will be amazed by how much more super life-giving oxygen fills your lungs as you practice *Bragg Super Power Breathing*.

Oxygen is one of the primary catalysts for energy and optimal health in the human body!

A raw food diet is highest in oxygen. Eat organic fresh fruits, green vegetables and sprouted seeds and nuts. Live fruits, green veggies and sprouted/soaked seeds and nuts are composed of water, which is composed of hydrogen and oxygen and mostly oxygen by weight. The green in vegetables is chlorophyll which is very close in its atomic structure to human blood. Chlorophyll has a magnesium atom and human blood differs only with an iron atom. With enzymes from raw food the magnesium ion is changed to an iron one making blood that can transport oxygen for human use instead of CO_2 for plant use.

An oxygen-depleting diet consists of cooked foods, red meat, sugar, saturated fats, white bread, processed and frozen foods, and carbonated beverages! Switching to an oxygen-rich diet often brings fast energy and a more vibrant body, skin and positive attitude! Choose foods rich in chlorophyll such as dark green leafy foods like spinach, collards, chard, kale, mustard greens, spirulina, chlorella and blue-green algae. Also try juicing them with veggies.

Adequate Hydration. Drinking enough water daily is essential not only for utilization of oxygen in the body, but also for transporting the blood and other bodily fluids. Without adequate water, all bodily functions are diminished, including cellular respiration and removal of toxins and metabolic wastes. Drinking 8 glasses of distilled water is necessary to get the full benefits of oxygenation.

Massage increases circulation which carries more oxygen to individual cells of the body. Massage enhances all essential body processes by opening the passageways of liquid and energy movement within the body.

Ozone air-purifying machines are extremely effective in destroying and eliminating airborne pollutants, fumes, cigarette smoke, odors, fungi, mold, bacteria, and viruses from the air.

The life-force and oxygen within me is feeding my strength – the strength of my body, soul and mind. – Paul C. Bragg, N.D., Ph.D.

Shallower, more rapid nervous breathing results in insufficient vital oxygen reaching the brain. – Susan Smith Jones, Ph.D., author "Health Bliss"

Your heart rate varies with your breathing: it slows down when you exhale and speeds up when you inhale. – Neil F. Gordon, author "Breathing Disorders"

Chapter 3

The Way You Breathe Affects Your Life

When you breathe deeply and more fully, you can live a healthier, happier, longer life.

When you pump a generous flow of oxygen into your body, every cell becomes more alive! This enables the four main *motors* of your body – the heart, lungs, liver and kidneys – to operate and perform better. Your miracle-working bloodstream purifies and cleanses every part of the body, including itself. This eliminates toxic wastes as Mother Nature planned. Then fuel (food) and vital oxygen are carried to every cell in your miracle body.

With ample oxygen your muscles, tendons and joints function more smoothly. Your skin becomes firmer and more resilient and your complexion clearer and glowing. You will radiate greater health, energy and well-being!

15

With Super Power Breathing your brain becomes more alert and your nervous system functions better. You become free from tension and strain because you can easily take the stresses and pressures of daily living. Your emotions come under your control. You feel joyous and exuberant. If negative emotions such as anger, hate, jealousy, greed or fear intrude, expel them with positive thinking and slow, concentrated, relaxed deep breathing!

The deep breather enjoys more peace of mind, tranquility and serenity! In India, the great teachers practice deep, full breathing as the first essential step towards higher spiritual development. You attain higher concentration in meditation by taking long, slow, deep breaths. Deep breathing stimulates your brain cells and promotes new brain cell growth.

I command my life force to breathe deeply for vibrant, super health. Oxygen is the vital, precious, invisible staff of life. – Paul C. Bragg, N.D., Ph.D.

Life is in the breath. He who half breathes, half lives! – Old Proverb

Super Deep Breathing Improves Your Brain

The person who breathes deeply and fully thinks more clearly and sharply! Oxygen stimulates your logic and intelligence. The more deeply and fully you breathe, the greater your power of concentration and the more your creative mind will assert itself. You will also develop greater extrasensory perception within your body, especially the brain. Scientists at the Salk Institute for Biological Studies, in La Jolla, CA, know that adults generate new brain cells in the hippocampus, an area in the brain which is responsible for learning and memory. Deep breathing nourishes and fine-tunes the brain and entire body!

Bragg Super Power Breathing will help to constantly rejuvenate you to a higher energy vibration of living! The more fully and deeply you breathe, the further you will travel to higher levels on the physical, mental and spiritual planes. **Now sit back, relax, close your eyes and for 3 to 5 minutes enjoy some slow, deep breathing!**

16

Correct Breathing Can Reduce Stress

Scientific studies have shown that correct breathing can help manage stress and stress-related conditions by soothing the autonomic nervous system. Deep breathing can help with a number of disorders, including: anxiety, asthma, Chronic Fatigue Syndrome, high blood pressure, insomnia, pain, panic attacks, eczema and stress.

When we breathe, the brain sets the breathing rate according to the carbon dioxide levels, rather than the oxygen levels. When a person is under stress, their breathing pattern changes. An anxious person takes small, shallow breaths, using their shoulders rather than their diaphragm to move the air in and out of their lungs. This can prolong feelings of anxiety and cause: headaches, fatigue, insomnia, chest tightness and muscle aches.

When a person is relaxed, their breathing is slower, more even and gentle. Relaxed breathing seems to calm the nervous system, which can lower the blood pressure and the heart rate, reduce stress hormones, improve the immune system, increase energy, and provide feelings of calm and well-being!

Proper Breathing Helps Control Emotions

Breathing is a necessity of life that usually occurs without much thought. When we are angry, fearful or anxious we tend to over-breathe or breathe too fast! When we experience sadness, suspense, conflict or depression, we tend to under-breathe or hold our breath. These changes are automatic without our deliberate effort to breathe. **When we deliberately think about our breathing we can use it to help calm our nervous system.**

While the negative emotions cause over-breathing or under-breathing, the positive emotions cause breathing to be deeper, easier and effortless! When we return our breathing to a deeper, smoother breath, we can reduce the strength of our negative emotions and restore more peace, serenity and happiness! You can start this process by taking ten deep, smooth, relaxing breaths. With each out breath, say the word "calm" or "relax" silently in your head and there you are relaxing! You have triggered a calming response! This is simple, effective and works!

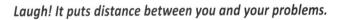

Start Being Happier, Smile & Laugh More – it's Up to You!

Healthy actions speak louder than words and can elevate your mood if you feel depressed. Take a brisk walk in a natural setting and practice slow, deep breathing – it helps you sort out and solve problems! Spend time with children, it simplifies life and puts everything in perspective. Find the comics in the newspaper or something funny to read and laugh. If someone is upset, try to analyze the situation from that person's perspective. As often as possible make yourself smile and laugh; it opens the blood vessels in the back of your head to physically lift your mood. Choose to be happy in spite of circumstances. No one "makes" you happy – it's an inner attitude that sparkles from within!

A laugh is just like sunshine. It freshens up the whole day. – Heart Warmers

---

Laughter is inner jogging, and good for your body and soul.
– Norman Cousins

Laugh! It puts distance between you and your problems.

Positive affirmations create miracles. – Beatrex Quntanna

A good laugh is sunshine in a house. – William Makepeace Thackeray

Super Power Breathing Calms the Nerves

The greatest tranquilizer for jangled nerves is deep, slow, diaphragmatic breathing. Today's tensions and pressures put additional strain on our nervous systems. The condition is aggravated by poor posture habits and shallow breathing. Your *Bragg Super Power Breathing Program* will help you correct both of these unhealthy habits . . . while having a calming, healthy effect on your nervous system and entire body!

During your workday, take a minute out of every hour to pause and s-t-r-e-t-c-h from your toes to the top of your head while doing deep, diaphragmatic breathing! Do back and forward shoulder rolls as well! The small amount of time invested in this program will pay dividends in productivity over the course of the day, because you will be able to work faster and with greater efficiency. This is especially important for those restricted to desks, but it's helpful in any kind of work. By oxygenating and relaxing your nerves, you will no longer be distracted or upset by petty annoyances at work or those minor irritations with fellow workers, family or friends.

18

Give Thanks to Your Miracle-Working Lungs

Every living thing breathes. Plants breathe through pores in their leaves. In the marvelous balance of Mother Nature, plants breathe in carbon dioxide and give off vital oxygen – while animals inhale oxygen and exhale carbon dioxide. Both thrive in a healthy, natural balance.

Unfortunately humans have played havoc with this natural balance by destroying forests and covering grass with pavement. They continue to poison our already over-burdened air with pollutants from motorized traffic and heavy industry. Wildlife, when it has survived slaughter by man, suffocates in such polluted air. Fish die in polluted waters. How long can people survive in the midst of the environmental poisons which they continually create? This is a question of great concern to us. Read the classic book *Silent Spring* by our friend Rachel Carson. If followed, her advice would have saved America and nations worldwide billions of dollars! We desperately need more courageous and dedicated people like Rachel Carson to show the world the error of its ways!

The Lower Respiratory System

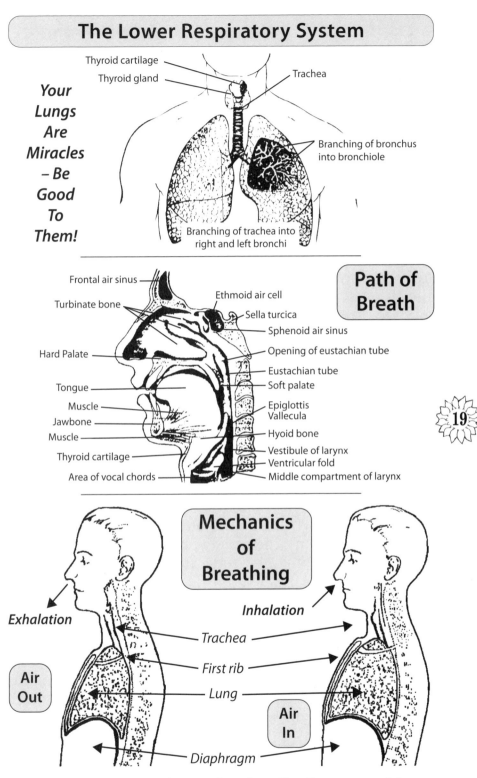

Your Lungs Are Miracles – Be Good To Them!

Thyroid cartilage
Thyroid gland
Trachea
Branching of bronchus into bronchiole
Branching of trachea into right and left bronchi

Path of Breath

Frontal air sinus
Turbinate bone
Ethmoid air cell
Sella turcica
Sphenoid air sinus
Hard Palate
Opening of eustachian tube
Eustachian tube
Tongue
Soft palate
Muscle
Epiglottis
Vallecula
Jawbone
Muscle
Hyoid bone
Thyroid cartilage
Vestibule of larynx
Ventricular fold
Area of vocal chords
Middle compartment of larynx

19

Mechanics of Breathing

Exhalation

Inhalation

Air Out

Trachea

First rib

Lung

Air In

Diaphragm

Mechanics of Breathing, showing diaphragm position and flexible ribs at exhalation and at inhalation.

The Lungs Are Nature's Miracle Breathers

Every animal in the world extracts oxygen from the environment in which it lives. Through their gills, fish extract oxygen from water (H_2O). Insects get oxygen from the air through alveoli or air cells in individual openings set in segments of their bodies. Worms and other invertebrates breathe through the pores of their skin.

Vertebrate animals including the human race, have those miracle mechanisms – the lungs. The mechanical equivalent would be a pair of bellows, though the lungs are superior and are far more intricate and adaptable.

Human lungs are a miraculous pair of conical-shaped organs composed of spongy, porous tissue. They occupy the thoracic cavity (chest) with the heart in the center, and are protected by the amazingly strong, flexible and resilient rib cage. The apex of each lung reaches just above the collar bone; the base extends to the waistline.

What makes up our lungs? About 300-500 million alveoli – air cells or sacs of elastic tissue – which can expand or contract like tiny balloons. If these little air sacs were flattened out and laid side by side, the flattened alveoli would cover an area the size of a tennis court. Tiny capillaries (blood vessels) thread elastic walls of each of the millions of air sacs, and it's through these that blood passes to remove its load of carbon dioxide that is expelled as we breathe out and then take in vital, life-giving oxygen. The average person has 5 to 6 quarts of blood, which must be continually cleansed.

Air inhaled through the nose and mouth reaches the alveoli through an intricate system of tubes, beginning with the large trachea, or windpipe, which is kept rigid by rings of cartilage in its walls. The trachea extends through the neck into the chest where it divides into two branches (bronchi), each leading into a lung cavity. Each bronchus divides into a number of successively smaller branches to bring air to every air sac. Your lungs are working miracles!

Man is composed of important elements as vital breath, deeds, thoughts and the senses. – The Upanishads

Success is deciding from the start what end result you want and creating the circumstances to realize and achieve that result. – Mark Victor Hansen

You Have Lungs – Fill Them Up

Each lung sits perfectly enveloped in a protective elastic membrane, the pleura, whose inner layer is attached to the lung and whose outer layer forms the lining of the thoracic cavity inside the rib cage. One end of each rib is attached to the spinal column, but the front of the rib cage is open. This allows lungs to expand and contract. When you breathe deeply, filling every air sac, your thoracic cavity expands as lungs breathe in about 500mL. This varies according to body build and size. Lung capacity (the maximum amount of air a person's lungs can hold) is about 4-6 liters.

This marvelous breathing mechanism is yours for free! You are born with it. It functions without conscious effort, yet without it, you cannot exist! **Start slow, deep relaxed breathing right now.**

Not even the latest medical inventions used by hospitals in emergencies, however ingenious, can equal your human breathing machine! Perhaps if human beings had to pay a fabulous price for their lungs and air, they would use them to full capacity all the time. Think of the big price you pay for only using them partially by shallow breathing. Remember, we are always only one breath away from death!

The Importance of Clean Air to Health

It is essential to breathe clean air – air that is as free as possible from such chemicals as smog, car exhaust, natural gas appliance fumes and many other toxic chemical pollutants. Our air also needs to be as free as possible from dust, dust mites and their fecal matter, animal dander, mold, and pollen. Everyone's health is helped in varying degrees by clean air! It's vitally important to live and work in an area which has clean air and that is free of all harmful fumes! It's also equally important to keep our homes pure, clean and free from clutter, dust and debris! **Most people cannot be truly 100% healthy and well until they breathe clean air, maintain a healthy diet and live a healthy lifestyle!**

Breathing is our connection to life, through the body & heart, leading us to a wholeness of being & giving us spirit for living life to its fullest. – S. Hainer, M.S.

On an average day your faithfully work lungs move enough air in and out to fill a medium-sized room or blow up several thousand party balloons.

Live Longer Breathing Clean Air Deeply

We advise those who live or work in smog-ridden, polluted cities to obtain a good air filter. We especially recommend filters which contain charcoal and a high efficiency particulate HEPA air filter. The charcoal removes most of the chemicals and the HEPA filter removes most of the particles. To be effective in an average room, the flow rate through the filter should be over 200 cubic feet of air per minute. The wise motorist will also install an air filter in his car for cleaning the air while driving in polluted cities.

When we are born, our lungs are new, fresh, clean, and rosy in color. If we could live in a dust-free atmosphere breathing deeply all our lives, then our lungs would remain *as good as new* for a long, healthy lifetime of use. Yet most people abuse their lungs! Some of this comes from external causes. The miracle lungs are the only organs of the body which are directly affected by external conditions, specifically, by the air we breathe into them!

Mother Nature has provided protection against a normal amount of dust contamination: tiny hairs in the nose serve as filters and moist mucus in the passages leading to the lungs trap dust particles that we expel through the nose or mouth. The tonsils also serve as guards to trap germs! The lungs protect themselves remarkably well by expelling carbon dioxide through oxygenation and by discharging toxins into the blood for elimination via the kidneys. **Your body is a miracle!**

Unfortunately, most civilized people today live in very unnatural conditions! There are abnormal amounts of pollutants in the air we breathe almost everywhere, especially in cities or populated areas. Our lungs are often overloaded with more contaminants than they can handle! These pollutants are passed along into the bloodstream and to other body parts. The lungs of modern city dwellers become brownish from car smog, soot, smoke, etc. Even in most farming areas, the lungs must contend with pollens, excessive dust, poisonous pesticides, fertilizers and other toxic chemicals.

Chapter 4

Smoking – A Deadly Habit That Destroys Lungs & Health

With all of these nearly inescapable health hazards and increased air pollution to overcome, it's incredible that millions of people harm their lungs even more by inhaling deadly tobacco smoke into their lungs daily.

Nicotine is poison! It immediately affects lung function. It constricts your cardiovascular system! It destroys vitamin C, which is vital to your health and immune system! After only 12 hours of not smoking, nicotine blood levels fall and the heart and lungs begin to start healing. If you smoke, please stop now and be loving to your body.

The lungs' air sacs are further damaged by tobacco tars and carbon particles. These lodge in the walls of the lungs' important balloon-like cells, causing them to lose their natural elasticity and eventually breaking them down altogether. The result? **Emphysema** – the killer disease in which the destruction of the breathing mechanism is sadly, slowly smothering and killing its victim from within!

23

Of the over 50 million Americans who smoke, one third to one half will die from smoking-related diseases! **Smoking also introduces two deadly poisons into the body: arsenic and carbon monoxide, as well as other toxins.** Compounding these health hazards, smoking creates an increased desire for caffeine and sugar. Moreover, twice as many smokers drink alcohol compared to non-smokers. Smokers have a far greater incidence of cancer of the lungs, larynx, pharynx, esophagus, mouth, colon and breast. **All tobacco products should be banned – they are killers!**

Data from the World Health Organization has found that deaths from lung cancer and chronic obstructive pulmonary disease (COPD) will rise over the next 20 years because of past smoking rates. It describes tobacco smoking as "the most important health hazard" and it maintains that smoking is the main preventable cause of death from lung cancer to coronary disease. – bbc.com/news/health

---

In China smoking is epidemic! Studies show that one-third of Chinese men will die of tobacco related diseases – sad facts!

Smoking and Your Lungs: What Cigarettes Do

When you smoke cigarettes, many chemicals enter your body through your lungs. Burning tobacco produces more than 4,000 chemicals. Nicotine, carbon monoxide, and tars are some of these substances. Smoking greatly affects your lungs and airways. Smokers get a variety of problems related to breathing ranging from an annoying cough to grave illnesses like emphysema and cancer.

How Your Lungs and Airways Change

Smoking causes many changes in your lungs and airways. Some changes are sudden, last a short time, and then go away. Other changes happen slowly and last a long time, often for the rest of your life. These are chronic changes. **Here is a list of some of the changes that happen in your lungs and airways when you smoke:**

- The cells that produce mucus in your lungs and airways grow. As a result, mucus increases and becomes thicker. Mucus stays in your airways, clogs them and makes you cough. This extra mucus can easily become infected.
- The lungs have broom-like hairs, called cilia, which clean your lungs. A few seconds after you start smoking, the cilia slow down. Smoking one cigarette can slow the action of your cilia for several hours and reduce the number of cilia, so there are fewer cilia to clean your lungs.
- Your lungs and airways get irritated and inflamed. They become narrow and reduce the air flow. Even one or two cigarettes can cause irritation and some coughing.
- When you smoke, your lungs age faster!!!
- Your lungs can be destroyed – the number of air spaces and blood vessels in the lungs decrease, then less much needed oxygen is carried to the rest of your body.
- When you smoke, the natural defenses your lungs have against infection are burdened and do not work well!
- Cigarette smoke has chemicals that can make normal cells change into cancer cells.

24

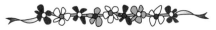

Please visit websites:
• www.cdc.gov/tobacco • BeTobaccoFree.hhs.gov • www.lung.org
for more info on smoking and damage it does to your lungs!

E-Cigarettes Are Not Healthy for You!

Electronic cigarette sales have grown to nearly $18.5 billion and continue to grow in the U.S. The popularity of these battery-operated nicotine inhalers are all the rage these days; however, much is still unknown about the health risks of E-Cigs or "vaping" as it is often called. What we do know is that it is banned in nearly a dozen countries, and the **World Health Organization is strongly against E-Cigarettes!**

Yet a New Zealand study said tobacco-free E-Cigs have proven as effective as nicotine patches at weaning smokers off their habit. Other specialists have said that E-Cigs have no tar build-up on the lungs as with traditional cigarettes nor are there trace chemicals that come from burning paper or tobacco. But in 2014 Japanese Researchers found harmful carcinogens and formaldehyde were present as well as hazardous chemicals including diethylene glycol, which is found in anti-freeze! Plus, Greek researchers found *E-Cigs increased breathing difficulties, while other studies have suggested that secondhand vapor poses health risks! The American Lung Association and other authorities assert that they are NOT safer than regular cigarettes!*

Wise Teens Talk About Stopping Smoking

Ex-smoking teens testify that their life is better, self-esteem higher and hope for the future more profound after they quit smoking! Often these misguided children begin smoking before they are old enough to appreciate their hard-working lungs! They begin filling their miracle breathing lungs with health destroying tobacco, some when they are 16, 14 and even 10 years old! Stan B. recalls, "I started smoking when I was 12, to look cool." Susan W. says, "I smoked two packs a day from the time I was 16."

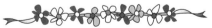

Your lungs are precious and needed every minute of your life. It's important to keep them clean and away from all smoke! – Patricia Bragg

ALL TOBACCO AND NICOTINE SHOULD BE BANNED – IT'S A KILLER! Shocking Sad Facts: Children and teenagers make up 90% of all the new smokers in United States. Sadly teenage and college smoking is on rise!

As horrifying as these shocking stories are, we can take heart from these youngsters and learn a lesson from their resiliency. Though they are young and the challenge they face is difficult, many teen smokers are winning the battle against their smoking habit, and feeling healthier and happier as a result! When it comes to quitting, Stan B. says, "It's not easy, I look at my parents who've smoked for 25 years! I know I don't want to be sucking smoke into my lungs and coughing like them."

Every smoking teen should remember that they are not alone in the struggle to quit, and that their goal is within reach. Many young adults now choose a healthy quality of life over one of the greatest destroyers of our time – smoking! And, should any smoking teen find themselves wavering in their efforts to quit, they should remember the words of ex-smoking teen Ann S., who explains, "The biggest reward was that my self-esteem became so much better – I don't need a cigarette to make everything okay. I enjoy a healthy lifestyle and have more money, time and energy!"

26 Quit Smoking – See the Difference it Makes!

• **20 MINUTES AFTER QUITTING:** Your blood pressure and pulse rate drop to normal. The temperature of your hands and feet increases to normal.

• **8 HOURS AFTER QUITTING:** The carbon monoxide level in your blood drops to normal. Amazingly, the life-giving oxygen level in your blood then increases to normal.

• **24 HOURS AFTER QUITTING:** You substantially lessen your chances of having a heart attack or stroke.

• **48 HOURS AFTER QUITTING:** Your nerve endings start regrowing and your ability to taste and smell is enhanced.

• **2 WEEKS TO 3 MONTHS AFTER QUITTING:** Your circulation improves. Brisk walking and exercise becomes easier. Your lung function increases and improves as much as 30 percent.

• **1 TO 9 MONTHS AFTER QUITTING:** Coughing, sinus congestion, fatigue and shortness of breath decreases. Your lungs and body are becoming cleaner and more resistant to infection.

• **1 YEAR AFTER QUITTING:** Excess risk for coronary heart disease decreases to an amazing 50% that of a smoker's.

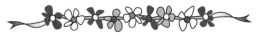

Smoking cigarettes is know to cause damage to every organ in your body. – CDC

- **2 TO 3 YEARS AFTER QUITTING:** The risk for coronary heart disease and stroke decrease to level of those who have never smoked. Also less of a chance of osteoporosis.
- **5 YEARS AFTER QUITTING:** Lung cancer death rate for the former one-pack-per-day smoker decreases by over half. Risks of mouth and throat cancer are half those of smokers.
- **10 TO 15 YEARS AFTER QUITTING:** Lung cancer death rate is almost that of non-smokers. Pre-cancerous cells are replaced. Risks for mouth, throat, esophagus, bladder, kidney, breast and pancreas cancer decrease. – *Prevention Magazine*

Deadly Smoking – A Health Hazard to Avoid – What it Does to You and Those Around You!

When people inhale deadly tobacco smoke into their miracle lungs, the protective cilia hairs filter out much of the smoke's harmful substances before it is exhaled. This means that while harmful toxins are trapped in the delicate linings of the smokers' lungs, fewer of these toxins are re-released into the air for others to breathe in. However, between a smoker's deadly puffs, the cigarette burns directly into the air. This smoke is known as "secondhand, side-stream" smoke, but it should be called "direct" smoke. Smoke that burns directly into the air is completely unfiltered and more deadly than the smokers' smoke! **Stay away from all deadly smoke!**

Recent studies establish that people who live or work around smokers are more likely to develop lung and sinus damage than smokers! For asthma or bronchitis sufferers, this exposure is very damaging. In addition to these dangers, "direct" smoke irritates the eyes, nose and throat and smells up everything it touches (rooms, hotels, offices, carpets, drapes, cars and everything around smoking).

There is good news. When a person stops smoking the cilia hairs begin to heal and move again. Smokers – stop now, you begin cleansing and healing immediately!

ONE EXCEPTION: A special blend of marijuana, for medicinal purposes, relieves pain in adults and stops seizures in children. – Dr. Sanjay Gupta

More than 40 million Americans are cigarette smokers. Nearly 70% of smokers report they want to quit, more than 42% say they've tried to quit during the past year. – CDC

DEADLY SMOKING FACTS!

✝ Tobacco use and also second-hand smoke will eventually kill over one fifth of world population – now more than 7 million yearly.

✝ Of the over 50 million Americans who smoke, one third to one half will die from a smoke-related disease and all will reduce their life expectancy by an average of nine years.

✝ Smoking acts as either a stimulant or a depressant – depending upon the smoker's emotional state at the time.

✝ The average pack-a-day smoker takes about 70,000 *hits* of deadly nicotine each year. Do visit and read: *www.ash.org*

✝ "Second hand smoke" hurts non-smokers: it speeds up their heart rate, raises blood pressure and doubles the amount of deadly carbon monoxide in their blood. It's a killer!

✝ Secondary deadly smoke contains more nicotine, tar and cadmium than mainstream smoke (leads to hypertension, emphysema, cancer, and asthma) and is killing millions!

✝ Babies born to mothers who smoke tend to have lower body weight, smaller lungs, poor health and many develop asthma.

✝ Lung illnesses are twice as common in smokers' children.

✝ Children and teenagers make up 90% of the new smokers in the United States – and teenage (deadly) smoking is on the rise!

✝ The death rate from breast cancer ranges from 25% to 75% higher among women who smoke. *www.BreastCancer.org*

✝ Female smokers may face a higher risk of lung cancer – as much as twice the risk of male smokers, according to a study done by Dr. Harvey Risch at Yale University.

✝ For both men and women, those who smoked more than two packs a day were 50 times more likely to develop lung cancer than those who never smoked (*National Cancer Institute*).

✝ Your body contains almost 100,000 miles of blood vessels. Smoking ages and constricts those vessels, depriving your body of important, rich oxygen it needs. Lack of oxygen causes serious illness.

✝ Tobacco is the main introduction to more deadly drugs!!!

✝ Teens who smoke are far more likely to engage in other risky and life-threatening behaviors (including using other dangerous drugs; violence; hatred; gang involvement; carrying weapons; and engaging in unprotected sex which often results in pregnancy or disease) than non-smoking healthy teens.

✝ Cataracts, cancer, angina, arteriosclerosis, osteoporosis, chronic bronchitis, asthma, high blood pressure, impotency and respiratory ailments are linked to all forms of smoking.

QUIT SMOKING! All smokers must stop this vicious, deadly smoking habit that destroys health, youth, energy and life!

Chapter 5

Common Cold – The Body's Miracle Cleansing Process

Any one day in winter, over 30 million Americans suffer with a bad cold. Adults average five to six colds per season, while children and teenagers often get double that amount. The body wants the toxins and mucus out!

Are these colds necessary? How do people *catch cold?* What causes the common cold? Medical Science has learned how to control many diseases that are far more serious, but remain baffled by the common cold. Is the culprit an unfiltered virus? Is it brought on by sitting in a draft, getting chilled, or getting one's feet wet, as is often suggested by mothers through the ages?

Colds Clean Out Mucus and Toxins

While the theories are many, there seems to be only one sure fact – people who are in perfect health don't generally *catch colds.* My dad spent a year living in the Arctic among the Eskimos. He never had a cold, and neither did they. He had the same experience in the South Seas, in the Balkans, among the nomads of the Middle East and with the native tribes of Africa. The common factor among all these people at the time was that they were breathing pure air, eating simple natural foods and getting plenty of exercise and sleep. By following this same basic healthy lifestyle, my Dad remained free of colds even in the midst of civilization.

Based on his research, he found that the *common cold* is Mother Nature's method of detoxifying the body. Most people are shallow breathers. And most live on an unhealthy diet of devitalized foods. Stress causes acidity, which leads to the body's inability to release toxins. Toxins start accumulating and clogging their bodies. That's why it's important to live a healthy lifestyle, plus incorporate some fasting.

29

Improved lung function guards against onset of illness.
– Holger Schunemann, M.D.

The Body Self-Cleanses, Repairs and Heals

When toxicity of accumulated poisons, mucus, environmental pollutants and stress exceed the body's tolerance, natural vital forces set up a miracle *cleansing-healing* (common colds) crisis. The body induces a rise in your body temperature (fever) to burn up the many toxins, while others are eliminated by heavy discharge of mucus from the nose, mouth and throat. If the toxic overload is heavy, there may be discharge of mucus from bowels and perhaps even diarrhea.

Instead of being alarmed, be grateful your body's natural Vital Forces are strong enough to take command by pushing out the toxins you have accumulated! Don't try to block this natural detox and healing process with antibiotics, aspirin, etc. Work with Mother Nature. Breathe deeply and fully to supply your body with the great purifier: oxygen. Rest and fast (page 141). Do a distilled water fast (8 glasses daily) or try a fresh juice fast (page 139). It's best to take only liquids during this cleansing and healing crisis. Your body will fight for its life against a great deal of abuse. When you follow Mother Nature's Laws and live The Bragg Healthy Lifestyle you can create a painless, tireless and ageless body. Miracles can happen!

Oxygen Cleanses and Nourishes

No germ can live in freshly squeezed organic orange juice because there is nothing in pure orange juice for it to feed on. All germs, regardless of their names, are scavengers! They feed on toxic decaying matter.

It's our personal opinion, based on experience and research, that a 100% healthy, natural foods diet – in combination with the enormous amount of pure oxygen pumped into the body by the vigorous breathing exercises taught in this book will help provide a natural immunity against most infectious diseases and germs.

Yogi Breathe Deep Organic Tea helps clear breathing passages and nourishes lung tissues. This healing formula utilizes licorice, basil, cinnamon, peppermint, ginger and herb thyme to loosen phlegm and relax muscles of respiratory tract.

Oxygen is not only the energizing factor which makes it possible for the body to eliminate putrefied matter on which germs thrive, it helps exterminate germs! As you deeply breathe more oxygen into your body and nourish it with organic, healthy foods, you give your body a greater ability to ward off germs and infections!

When we practice Super Power Breathing, we increase our cardiovascular respiratory power! We purify and energize our bloodstream to carry more powerful, revitalizing oxygen to the heart and entire cardiovascular system. Start practicing today – you will benefit greatly.

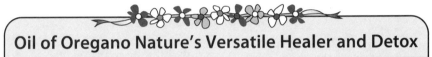

Oil of Oregano Nature's Versatile Healer and Detox

Oil of Oregano: is a powerful herbal body defender and cleanser and is used to fight: viruses; flus; colds; allergies; asthma; E. coli; Salmonella; parasitic yeast and bacterial infections; upset stomach; menstrual problems; urinary tract problems and arthritis. Take with food. Available in caps or drops at Health and Vitamin Stores. (When needed for winter cold maintenance use caps and drops, and do the Breathing Detox below.)

Helpful Breathing Detox: Place 2-3 drops of *Oil of Oregano* in two quarts of boiling water. Put a towel over your head, breathe in the vapors through your mouth, then your nose. It's powerful – close your eyes! This opens up the lungs to remove congestion. Relieves colds, flu, bronchitis and congestion. Do as needed one to three times daily. Also try 1 drop of oil in juice.

"When you feel a cold or any illness coming on, or are just depressed – it is best to fast! Each time you fast, you will feel better. Your body will then have a chance to cleanse and heal and rebuild its immune system by regular fasting. Bragg Health Books were my conversion to the healthy way. Everyone should read Bragg's 'Miracle of Fasting' book!" (see back pages for Bragg booklist)
– James Balch, M.D., co-author "Prescription for Nutritional Healing"

Whatever occurs in the mind, effects the body and visa versa. Mind and body cannot be considered independently. When the two are out of sync, both emotional and physical stress can erupt.
– Hippocrates, Father of Medicine, 400 B.C.

Life is a precious, beautiful song and love is the music.

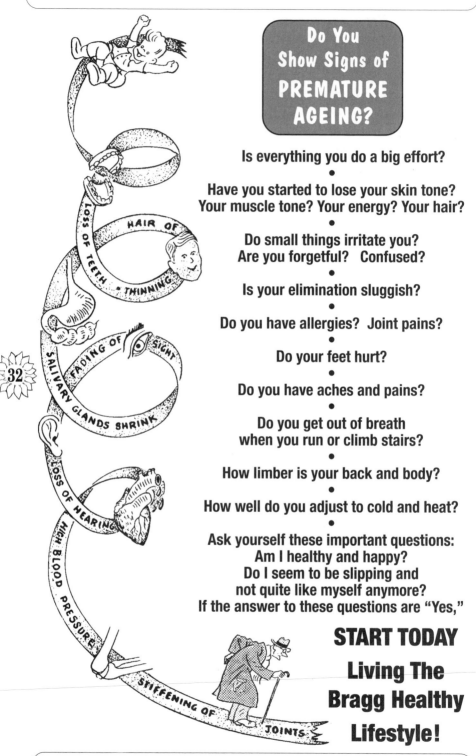

Do You Show Signs of PREMATURE AGEING?

Is everything you do a big effort?

•

Have you started to lose your skin tone?
Your muscle tone? Your energy? Your hair?

•

Do small things irritate you?
Are you forgetful?   Confused?

•

Is your elimination sluggish?

•

Do you have allergies? Joint pains?

•

Do your feet hurt?

•

Do you have aches and pains?

•

Do you get out of breath
when you run or climb stairs?

•

How limber is your back and body?

•

How well do you adjust to cold and heat?

•

Ask yourself these important questions:
Am I healthy and happy?
Do I seem to be slipping and
not quite like myself anymore?
If the answer to these questions are "Yes,"

START TODAY
Living The
Bragg Healthy
Lifestyle!

He who understands and follows Mother Nature walks with God.

Chapter 6

Your Miracle Nose – Pathway to the Lungs

The Bragg Super Power Breathing technique is the most essential part of The Bragg Healthy Lifestyle. Your nose and nasal passageways are essential factors in all your breathing. So it's important that we understand the nose and the vital health role it plays in breathing.

The nose is a system of passages and hollow spaces that link the external nose to the eyes, ears, mouth and throat. It is through this intricate pathway that oxygen-rich air travels from our nose to our lungs. You might wonder why we have all this complicated breathing mechanism made up of cartilage, bone, and soft tissue organized into several pairs of hollow air-spaces called sinuses. When afflicted with some sinus or nasal complaint you might think it just can't be worth all the trouble. After all, the mouth and throat seem to **33** do the breathing work just fine – and it's just a simple and direct air pathway to the lungs.

We Mostly Breathe Through the Nose

We do most breathing through the nose. That means that the oxygen required to nourish our bodies moves through the nose 22,000 or more times a day, depending upon whether you are a shallow, deep or slow breather. So then, why is this part of our body so complex and a site of so many health complaints? The answer is that the nose is a lot more than just a pathway for air to get to the lungs, it's a miracle-working part of your body!

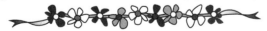

Shallow breathing helps to increase symptoms of almost every known sickness!

The quality of the blood depends largely upon its oxygenation in the lungs.
– Basic Physiology

 What a person eats becomes his own body chemistry.
– Paul C. Bragg, N.D., Ph.D., Originator of Health Stores

Your Nose is a Miracle Air-Filtration System

The hollow spaces of the nose – called sinuses – act as "echo chambers" (eight *air pockets*), which make our voices resonate (unless sinuses are stuffed up). These open spaces (located behind our eyebrows, nose, cheeks, and between the eyes) also give us better balance and cushion the brain from blows to the head. Our sense of smell is located in the nose. The most important function of the nose, the sinuses and nose hairs, is to condition and filter the air as it passes through to your faithful, hard-working lungs.

The membranes of the nose and sinuses produce between a pint and a quart of mucus every day. These secretions line the walls of the nose and sinuses and are always on the move. As the mucus passes through the sinus cavities, it collects dust particles, bacteria and other air pollutants that were breathed in along with the oxygen-rich air that nourishes every corner of the body. These same airways are lined with little filter hairs (called *cilia*) which strongly try to keep out all dust and pollutants from the air we breathe.

It's the nose that tries its best to protect the lungs and all your body cells from any airborne pollutants and contaminants! Under healthy conditions, our lungs receive clean air even with some pollution, thanks to our nose filters! Sadly, in the world many areas have heavy pollution that plagues our air and takes its toll on the health of the body! The nose takes the brunt of the attack, then lungs and the body.

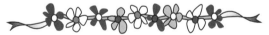

BRONCHIAL DRAINAGE: Use gravity to move secretions and mucus from small airways into larger ones and out for easier breathing. All positions are done with head lower than hips on a slant or incline board. You can try laying on your back, stomach or sides. Try each position 5-15 minutes.

The body is self-cleansing and self-healing when you give it a chance with a fasting detox cleanse and living a healthy lifestyle!
– Patricia Bragg

Your body wants mucus and toxic slime out! Do all you can to help remove these toxins. When you feel them in your throat and sinuses, cough, spit and blow the mucus out. – The Bragg Healthy Lifestyle book

Sinusitis Causes Breathing & Infection Problems

Sinus complaints usually are signs of the nose trying to do its job of protecting the lungs in troubled times. The nasal passages can suffer from the contaminants they work hard to block. Sometimes the sinuses become irritated or inflamed from air pollution, smoke, mold, pet dander, infection, or an allergy attack (for most common food allergies see page 38) brought on by some of these irritating toxic factors.

Blocked Sinuses Breed Health Problems

When the nose and sinuses become over-burdened, they secrete mucus and swell. This blocks the openings and prevents the flow of mucus and air. This causes a breathing problem that creates an environment where bacteria can flourish. This unhealthy situation weakens the nose and sets the stage for sinus and asthma problems, poor breathing and infections, etc.

Many people who suffer from blocked and painful sinuses run to the drug store for over-the-counter medical relief. They hope nasal sprays will relieve their breathing problems. Many don't follow directions and abuse the sprays, often becoming addicted with disastrous consequences. Forcing sinuses open continually can cause harm, because they close up to protect lungs from airborne toxins, etc. "If your sinuses are the problem, longer use puts you at risk for a chronic situation of diminishing returns," says Joel Saper, M.D.

Nasal spray abuse can also cause a secondary illness, *rhinitis medicamentosa,* when the nose becomes inflamed by the medicine itself. Instead of quick-fix relief of a drug, take a long-term view of your nose's health. Remember, your nose is the pathway to your lungs, and the point of entry for the body's most needed, elemental nutrient – oxygen. Your nose deserves to be treated with loving, gentle care!

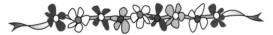

A large percent of sinus problems are caused by bacteria, pollutants, such as smoke and dust, allergies and overuse of nasal decongestant medication.

Other Healthy Ways to Unblock Your Sinuses

Herbs (tea or capsules): fenugreek, echinacea, anise, marshmallow and red clover, help to loosen phlegm and clear congestion; rosehips, horehound and mullein help relieve symptoms. Golden Seal: an anti-microbial and immune booster herb is also beneficial for respiratory conditions. Ginger is another herb you can use by steeping thin slices in hot water for 10 minutes, then drink it as tea. Inhaling warm vapors can also relieve pain and pressure.

Inhale eucalyptus, lavender, peppermint or basil oils: put a few drops in boiling water, turn the heat off, put a towel over your head and carefully breathe the vapors.

Drink 8 or more glasses distilled water daily: You can add raw, organic apple cider vinegar to three of them – see recipe on page 144.

Solve Sinus and Allergy Problems

36 For a healthy nose, it's essential you live The Bragg Healthy Lifestyle. A balanced, healthy life is the basis for good health! A healthy, happy head and body are necessary preconditions to a healthy nose. If you live in a polluted area, smokers, etc. or if sinuses are already damaged from the hard work of protecting your lungs, buy a high-efficiency HEPA (microscopic pores remove almost all particles) air filtration system. This pre-filters and cleans the air you breathe, making the job easier for your nose. Also enjoy herbal teas (see above) or take them in capsule form. You must be intelligent about allergies. If you know you're allergic to particular substances, take precautions to avoid them. If you suspect allergies, take all necessary steps to learn if and what you are allergic to. The most common allergens are mold

Apple Cider Vinegar, Lemon & Cayenne Pepper Cold Remedy

Try out this strange and spicy brew and find some relief! 4 Tbsps. each of water and organic, raw apple cider vinegar, 1 Tbsp. honey, 1/8 tsp. cayenne pepper and 1 wedge of lemon. Bring water to a boil. Combine water and ACV in a small glass or mug. Add honey and cayenne pepper. Stir well. Add squeeze of lemon. Start drinking.

spores, animal dandruff, and house dust. Also, food allergies (see chart page 38) are high sources of allergic reactions; they are associated with the nose, sinus, and mucus complaints.

It is of utmost importance to avoid dairy products. Millions suffer allergic reactions (mucus, colds, etc.) to dairy products because they are very unhealthy for the nose and the whole body. Dairy proteins can cause the nose and throat airway passages to swell. They also produce mucus-causing sinus discomfort and bacterial mucus conditions. If you snore (page 96-97) or suffer a sinus problem, a non-dairy diet brings miracle improvements!

Read these two important books on milk and why it is best to avoid:

- *Mad Cows and Milk Gate* by Virgil Hulse M.D.
- *Milk, the Deadly Poison* by Robert Cohen

Also visit these websites:

- *www.notmilk.com* • *pcrm.org*

(Physicians Committee for Responsible Medicine)

Allergies, Daily Journal & Dr. Coca's Pulse Test

Almost every known food may cause some allergic reaction at times. Thus, foods used in *elimination diets* may cause allergic reactions in some individuals. Some are listed among the **Most Common Food Allergies** (see next page). Since reaction to these foods is generally low, they are widely used in making test diets. By keeping a food journal and tracking your pulse rate after meals you will soon know your problem foods. Allergic foods cause pulse rate to go up. (Take base pulse, for 1 minute, before meals, then 30 minutes after meals, and also before bed. If it increases 8-10 beats per minute – check foods for allergies.)

Your nose is the only organ able to properly prepare the air you breathe.
Mouth breathing and resultant over-breathing elevates your blood pressure
and heart rate and worsens asthma, allergies, rhinitis, sleep apnea, and
deprives your heart, brain and other organs of optimal oxygenation.
– Breathing.com

If your body has a reaction after eating some particular food, especially if it happens each time you eat that food, you may have an allergy. Some allergic reactions are: wheezing, sneezing, stuffy nose, nasal drip or mucus, dark circles, eye watering or waterbags under eyes, headaches, feeling light-headed or dizzy, fast heart beat, stomach or chest pains, diarrhea, extreme thirst, breaking out in a rash, swelling of extremities or stomach bloating, etc. (Read Dr. Arthur Coca's book, *The Pulse Test.*)

If you know what you're allergic to, you are lucky; if you don't, you had better find out as fast as possible and eliminate all irritating foods from your diet. To re-evaluate your daily life and have a health guide to your future, start a daily journal (copy page 146) of foods eaten, your pulse rate before and after meals and your reactions, moods, energy levels, weight, elimination and sleep patterns. You will discover the foods and situations causing problems. By charting your diet you will be amazed at the effects of eating certain foods. We have kept daily journals for years.

If you are hypersensitive to certain foods, you must omit them from your diet! There are hundreds of allergies and of course it's impossible here to take up each one. Many have allergies to milk, wheat, or some are allergic to all grains. Visit web: *FoodAllergy.org.* Your daily journal will help you discover and accurately pinpoint the foods and situations causing you problems. Start your journal today!

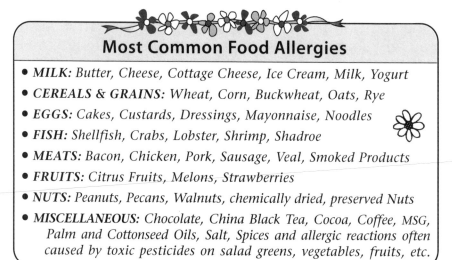

Most Common Food Allergies

- **MILK:** *Butter, Cheese, Cottage Cheese, Ice Cream, Milk, Yogurt*
- **CEREALS & GRAINS:** *Wheat, Corn, Buckwheat, Oats, Rye*
- **EGGS:** *Cakes, Custards, Dressings, Mayonnaise, Noodles*
- **FISH:** *Shellfish, Crabs, Lobster, Shrimp, Shadroe*
- **MEATS:** *Bacon, Chicken, Pork, Sausage, Veal, Smoked Products*
- **FRUITS:** *Citrus Fruits, Melons, Strawberries*
- **NUTS:** *Peanuts, Pecans, Walnuts, chemically dried, preserved Nuts*
- **MISCELLANEOUS:** *Chocolate, China Black Tea, Cocoa, Coffee, MSG, Palm and Cottonseed Oils, Salt, Spices and allergic reactions often caused by toxic pesticides on salad greens, vegetables, fruits, etc.*

Take Precautions to Prevent Nosebleeds

Another common health complaint is nosebleeds. Various conditions cause nosebleeds, including blows to face, excessive dryness, changes in atmospheric pressure, and scratching or blowing the nose too strenuously.

Nosebleeds can be classified either as anterior (discharging out the nose) or posterior (discharging down the throat). Posterior bleeding originates in the sinus cavities behind the eyebrows, nose or between the eyes. No matter what position the person is in, blood will drain out the back of the mouth and down the throat. This condition can affect the elderly that have high blood pressure. The anterior nosebleed is a common variety and flows out of the nostrils – although if one lies down, the blood may flow down the throat. Rarely serious, it can usually be treated by applying pressure to the nose and ice to the injured area. (Soak cotton ball in apple cider vinegar, lightly pack in the nostril and press – this can help blood to coagulate.)

Because excessively dry air can cause nasal membranes to crack, form crusts and bleed, increase the humidity in your house if you reside in a dry climate. You can do this with a commercial humidifier. If you need a quick fix, place a pan of boiling water in a small room. To help alleviate dry, sore nasal membranes, nightly gently pat aloe-vera, vitamin E, olive oil or comfrey ointment inside your nose.

Nosebleeds might be caused by a vitamin K deficiency. This is a crucial mineral for normal blood clotting. If you don't have your fair share, your nose will be more likely to bleed at the least provocation. You can remedy this situation by practicing wise, healthy, natural eating habits. The best vitamin K sources include sprouts, all dark-green leafy vegetables, sea greens, oats, eggs, molasses, alfalfa, wheatgrass, barley and spirulina.

Vitamin K helps to prevent hardening of the arteries, which is a common factor in coronary disease and heart failure. Research suggests vitamin K may help to keep calcium out of your artery linings and other body tissues, where it can cause damage. The latest studies show Vitamin K with vitamin D, prevents calcification in your coronary arteries, thereby preventing heart disease.

Exercise and Eat for Total Health

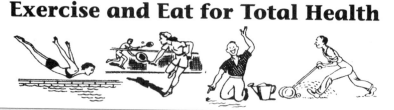

Enjoy Bragg Healthy Lifestyle
For a Lifetime of Super Health

In a broad sense, The Bragg Healthy Lifestyle for the Total Person is a combination of physical, mental, emotional, social and spiritual components. The ability of the individual to function effectively in his environment depends on how smoothly these components function as a whole. Of all the qualities that comprise an integrated personality, a totally healthy, fit body is one of the most desirable . . . so start today to achieve your health goals!

A person may be said to be totally physically fit if he functions as a total personality with efficiency and without pain or discomfort of any kind. This is to have a painless, tireless, ageless body. One possessing sufficient muscular strength and endurance to maintain a healthy posture and successfully carry on the duties imposed by life and the environment. To be able to handle emergencies and have enough energy for recreation and social obligations after the "work day" has ended. It is to meet the requirements of his environment through possessing the resilience to recover rapidly from fatigue, tension, stress and strain of daily living without the aid of stimulants, drugs or alcohol. To be able to enjoy natural recharging sleep at night and awaken fit and alert in the morning for the challenges of the new fresh day ahead.

Keeping the body totally healthy and fit is not a job for the uninformed or the careless person. It requires an understanding of the body and of a healthy lifestyle and then following it for a long, happy lifetime of health! The result of "The Bragg Healthy Lifestyle" is to wake up the possibilities within you, rejuvenate your body, mind and soul to total balanced health. It's within your reach, so don't procrastinate, start today! Our hearts and prayers go out to touch you with nourishing, caring love for your total health and life!

Patricia Bragg and *Paul C. Bragg*

Chapter 7

Your Diaphragm – The Key to Bragg Super Power Breathing

What is our secret of deep Super Power Breathing? How can you draw air into the very base of your lungs? Not by merely sniffing it in through your nose nor by gasping it in through your mouth!

Babies breathe naturally by using their diaphragms to create suction which pulls air into the lungs. Air may enter the body through either the nose or the mouth. But the pulling force which draws the air in, filling the air sacs of the lungs to capacity, comes from the strong muscular action of the powerful diaphragm.

The miracle diaphragm is a dome-shaped sheet of strong muscle fibers. It separates the thoracic (upper) half of your body, which contains the heart and lungs – from the abdominal (lower) cavity, which houses the organs of digestion and elimination. The diaphragm stretches from the sternum (breastbone) in front and across the bottom of the ribs to the backbone.

As the diaphragm expands and flattens, it then moves downward, producing suction within the chest cavity and pulling air into the lungs (inhalation). When the diaphragm relaxes and rises, it forces air out of the lungs (exhalation). Both operations are equally important: inhalation to bring in life-giving oxygen; exhalation to expel all of the collected poisonous carbon dioxide.

Before you can take a deep breath, you have to give one away. Why? Because, when you've been breathing in a shallow manner (from your chest), if you try and take a deep inhale, you just can't do it. All you can do is take a more labored, shallow breath from your chest. Slow, deep breathing out, and then breathing in, a full deep breath – works miracles! – See web: AnxietyCoach.com

During times of stress and anger, we tend to inhale and hold our breath. The most significant, therapeutic aspect of diaphragmatic breathing is the exhalation – which is best at least two times the length of the inhalation. The slow exhalation alerts the body that it can relax and resume essential body functions and not remain in state of upset, fight or flight. – Paul C. Bragg

Diaphragmatic Versus Chest Breathing

Chest breathing results from the movement of the rib section of the trunk, especially the upper section of the chest. When a person inhales, the chest expands, becoming larger. When he exhales, the chest relaxes, and then becomes smaller. When performed to the limit of inhalation and exhalation, it's an excellent form of internal exercise that helps the whole waist area and internal organs. It also develops the chest and has many other health benefits.

A great deal is made about *chest expansion* . . . the number of inches which the chest expands from a relaxed position (after exhalation) to that when the lungs are filled with air. However, people with large chests breathe no more effectively than those people with average-sized chests who use their breathing organs efficiently to spread oxygen throughout their bodies.

Chest Breathing: the body undertakes this natural method only during strenuous exertion. It might be termed a form of *forced breathing*. It is an emergency measure. Unfortunately, most people rob themselves of oxygen when they breathe, because they use only a minimum of the top portion of their lungs.

Diaphragmatic Breathing: this is the natural method designed for the body. When you inhale, the diaphragm expands. It not only expands the chest cavity and draws air into the lungs, but it also expands the abdominal cavity. It does more than just drawing in air, it stretches and massages the abdominal muscles and organs. When you exhale the diaphragm relaxes. It expels air from the lungs, exercises the rib muscles and massages the heart. Because this tones and tightens the abdominal muscles, you get healthier with each super power breath!

Wake up and say, "Today I am going to be happier, healthier and wiser in my daily living. I am the captain of my life and am going to steer it for 100% healthy lifestyle living!" Fact: Happy people look younger, have fewer health problems and live longer! – Patricia Bragg, Pioneer Health Crusader

---

Harmonious, rhythmic breathing massages the heart, liver and pancreas, and helps improve functions of the spleen, stomach, small intestine and abdomen. Your nerves will be calm, your voice will relax and your face will shine with a soft, healthy glow.

Internal Massage by Diaphragmatic Action

The diaphragm's effect on the muscles and organs of the abdomen is highly beneficial. To combat the pull of gravity and hold the abdominal organs in place, our abdominal muscles need all the exercise we can find time to give them. Correct, natural diaphragmatic breathing – along with daily exercise and practicing good posture (pages 161-168) – helps to accomplish many health miracles.

Your diaphragmatic natural action also provides an important massage for the heart, chest and stomach areas, as well as the liver, intestines, kidneys, gallbladder, spleen and pancreas. This stimulates blood circulation and helps these organs to perform the functions which are essential to maintaining your health for a long life!

The dual action of the diaphragm, which affects the upper thoracic organs (heart and lungs) and the lower abdominal organs, is a vital factor in good blood circulation. This is especially true as blood returns through the veins to the heart. The forceful pumping thrust of the heart muscles sends blood coursing through the arteries. This force is almost spent by the time the bloodstream has dispensed oxygen, nutrients and collected wastes, and is ready to return to the heart through the veins. The return trip is dependent upon the contraction of the muscles and muscular walls of the viscera – the internal organs contained within the abdominal and thoracic cavities. The rhythmic massage of the abdominal organs by the respiratory muscles plays a pivotal role in this vital return of blood to the heart.

Diaphragmatic breathing stimulates the *peristalsis,* the wavelike-squeezing motion of the intestines which promotes digestion and the elimination of solid and semi-solid fecal wastes. Making a change from chest breathing to diaphragmatic breathing has helped thousands in correcting heartburn, indigestion, gas, chronic constipation, liver problems, etc.

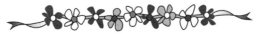

Deep Healthy Breathing: is about 10-12 breaths per minute, from the diaphragm (rather than the chest), through the nose (rather than mouth) and is quiet and light. Deep breathing techniques increase oxygenation!
– Mike Adams, Health Ranger

Bragg Super Power Breathing Calms the Nervous System

The *solar plexus* is the *powerhouse* of the body. It's a network of nerves and ganglia (independent groups of nerve cells) which control every vital organ in the abdominal cavity and is located in the center of the diaphragm. The more stimulation you give your diaphragm, the more circulation your solar plexus (often called the gut) receives. This increases the amount of nerve energy that is available to your vital organs. The extremely important pneumogastric nerve (*pneuma* – lungs; *gastro* – stomach) passes through the diaphragm and also benefits from this diaphragmatic action.

Diaphragmatic breathing has a tranquilizing rhythm, stimulates your circulation and helps rejuvenate the body. B-complex vitamins also have a calming effect on the entire nervous system. Diaphragmatic breathing breaks up the paralyzing nerve tension so often observed in people with supersensitive or jangled nerves. For more details about the beneficial effects of deep breathing on the nerves, read our book *Building Powerful Nerve Force & Positive Energy*.

44

Yoga teaches that deep, rhythmic breathing attunes one to the *rhythm of the universe* – in other words, one lives in rhythmic harmony with Mother Nature. *Prana*, the Sanskrit word for *breath*, also means *absolute energy* or *vital cosmic energy*. According to the teachings of yoga, when we breathe correctly we store this energy in the solar plexus.

The Ayurvedic Health and Fitness Lifestyle

An ancient healing system developed in India many thousands of years ago, Ayurveda (means science of life) offers therapies for health and fitness, along with yoga and herbs. In the ancient teachings of Ayurveda, a person's mind-body type is determined, then specific diet, exercise and lifestyle routines are prescribed that are best for them, according to their mind and body type.

You are where you are because you want to be there. If you want to be somewhere else, you'll need to change. – Mark Victor Hansen, co-producer, "Chicken Soup for the Soul" Series

---

I strive to be pure and good in all things – in body, mind & soul. – Paul C. Bragg

Ancient Yoga Breathing Promotes Health

Essential to Ayurveda is the daily practice of yoga stretching and the importance of breathing correctly. Yoga breathing helps the mind and body become one. Learning to breathe correctly helps you remain calm in your daily living, during exercise and in stressful times.

Yoga breathing is nose breathing. For centuries, this has been known to slow the heart, lower blood pressure and relieve stress. Because it is a more efficient way to get oxygen into your body, it will enhance athletic performance. To practice it, start by doing some yoga stretches. Then walk with gradually increasing speed – breathing only through your nose – until you are jogging. When you can no longer nose-breathe easily, slow down until you can again breathe comfortably through your nose. Do this back and forth several times – jogging and/or walking, always breathing through your nose. Finish with enjoyable yoga stretches. Practiced regularly, this calms you and gives you a greater oxygen capacity intake and increased energy, health and vitality. See website: *www.HealthAndYoga.com.*

45

The Benefits of Full Yoga Breathing

- Releases acute and chronic muscular tensions in the body, especially around the heart and digestive organs.
- Increases lung capacity – this helps asthma and emphysema sufferers overcome their fear of having shortness of breath attacks.
- Encourages proper nervous stimulus to the cardio-vascular system.
- Dramatically reduces emotional and nervous anxiety.
- Improves detox by increased carbon dioxide and oxygen exchange.
- Helps auto immune system by increased energy to endocrine system that regulates metabolism, tissue function, internal temperature, water balance, ions and moods.
- Calms the mind and integrates the mental and physical balance.
- Contributes to both vitality, energy, and relaxation.

With such powerful all-round benefits, do you really need to be "motivated" to get going? Take charge of your life! – *HealthAndYoga.com*

THE BREATH BUILDER®: An exercise tool for anyone who recognizes the value of deep breathing. Used regularly, the Breath Builder exerciser will increase the amount of air you inhale and exhale. It can benefit anyone . . . but especially helpful for persons suffering from emphysema or any other breathing problems. The Breath Builder will bring new life to the body, new energy to the spirit and new gusto to living! Available: www.stretching.com

No One Can Breathe for You

You can build a new figure, a new "you" – inside and out – vibrant, healthy and tingling with the joy of life. Remember, "you and you alone have this great power to breathe deeply – you are your captain, it's all up to you!"

This self-power to breathe deeply has no value unless it is used every day. You can build better blood circulation by daily doing The Bragg Super Power Breathing exercises and living The Bragg Healthy Lifestyle. You will soon become oxygen recharged and not feel fatigued at the least physical effort. Prove this to yourself – start today!

Breathing exercises bring sparkle to your eyes, a glow to your flesh and add vim and vigor to your step. You will be more mentally alert. Your reflexes will function better. You will feel more fit with a sense of well-being that is a far greater treasure than any material possession!

Oxygen is the most valuable of all nature's elements and you can have all you can breathe for free. You have only to learn how to fully utilize it with Bragg Super Power Breathing. By practicing long, slow breathing and taking longer, deeper breaths per minute you will enjoy greater health, more endurance, vitality, energy and a youthful life!

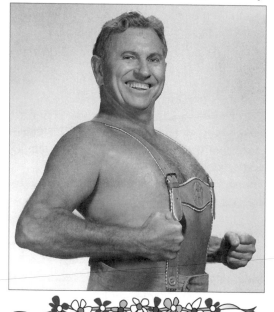

Breathing deeply gives you more energy, go-power and sparkles up your life!
– Paul C. Bragg, N.D., Ph.D., Health Crusader & Lifestyle Educator

46

Chapter 8

Super Power Breathing –
Your Way to Health & Happiness

Your lungs can hold at least six pints of air. If you keep your lungs filled to capacity you will feel better, have more energy, suffer less fatigue, sleep better, wake up refreshed and be a healthier, happier person. With practice you can easily learn to control your breathing, taking only 6 to 8 long, full breaths per minute for a healthier and more energized productive life. Start now!

Super Oxygen Breathing for Super Living

When your body is fed with Live Foods and Super Oxygen, the joy of living will thrill you. Every day you bounce out of bed with a glad to be alive feeling, knowing there is meaning in life. You'll have fewer depressing thoughts, and less anger, fewer frustrations, fears, or worries!

With the stimulation of Super Oxygen, you are eager to meet life's problems. You meet them face to face and find solutions. You enjoy the effort of facing life's realities.

47

Deep Breathing and Walk Worries Away!

You can truly *walk your worries away!* As the blood (*your river of life*) courses through your arteries and veins, cleansing and nourishing your entire body, you become filled with a sense of well-being. This cleanses your mind of its troubles and nourishes it with positive, healthy, happy thoughts.

Look at your life. Has it become overly complex? Have you found yourself burdened by too many possessions or responsibilities? Take a slow, deep breath and ask: "What steps can I take to reduce clutter so I may live life simply and joyously?" – Douglas Bloch, M.A., author, teacher and counselor

---

We are a product of our thoughts – and so is our health! While doctors and medicine have their place, self-healing is the most powerful medicine of all. Accepting the present and placing trust in a higher power frees your energy to focus on improving your life! See problems as challenges of growth, not as a punishment or judgement! Focus on happiness, forgiveness, hope and peace of mind, as well as physical change to ease any problems and situations.

Enjoy your walk with a free spirit and a light heart. Start at your own pace to fit the movement – fast, medium or slow. Watch with interest the things and people you pass, or let your walking be an accompaniment to your ideas and thoughts. As you breathe and walk rhythmically, awareness of your body will diminish. You will become more at peace and happier and in tune with Mother Earth.

As we stride along on our brisk walks we say, "Health, Strength, Youth, Vitality, Peace, Love, Joy, Eternity!" With walking you discover the beauty of God and Mother Nature as it awakens, softens and enriches your soul and life!

Deep Breathing Key to Healthy, Happy Life!

Health and happiness may reside in your brain, and more specifically with the power of your breath. You may be surprised to learn that advances and studies in "mind-body medicine" offer a deeper understanding of how something as simple as your breath could be the answer to your health, happiness and longevity!

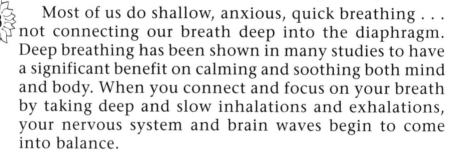

Most of us do shallow, anxious, quick breathing . . . not connecting our breath deep into the diaphragm. Deep breathing has been shown in many studies to have a significant benefit on calming and soothing both mind and body. When you connect and focus on your breath by taking deep and slow inhalations and exhalations, your nervous system and brain waves begin to come into balance.

Many ancient healing traditions, such as Yoga, meditation and Tai Chi, have recognized that one of the simplest and most effective tools we have to create more happiness in our life is to do deep breathing exercises. Medical studies suggest that deep, conscious, breathing might have the same effects as anti-depressant medication! Info from web: *www.DrJayKumar.com*

Some of life's greatest pleasures happen when we slow down, and enjoy the little things that brighten life. – Mac Anderson

---

The health of people is really the foundation upon which all their happiness and all their powers as a state depend.
– Benjamin Disraeli, former UK Prime Minister

Can Deep Breathing Influence Your Happiness?

Deep breathing engages the diaphragm, the muscle which divides your chest from your abdomen. On an inhale, the diaphragm moves down to allow the lungs to expand with oxygen. On the exhale, the diaphragm presses up against the lungs to dispel carbon dioxide.

Most of us slip into the habit of breathing with the upper half of our lungs. Our intercostal muscles get a workout, but our belly barely moves. Inside the chest, this means the lower lobes of our lungs don't get a full helping of fresh oxygen. According to Harvard Medical School, many small blood vessels instrumental in carrying oxygen to cells reside in the lowest portion of the lungs. When these areas are deprived of air, you can feel short of breath and anxious – which is the opposite of feeling happy.

Deep breathing stimulates the parasympathetic nervous system, which guides the body from stress to relaxation. When we're relaxed, our heart rate and blood pressure lowers, and our digestion and health improves.

49

By training yourself to breathe slowly and deeply in your everyday life, you're priming your body to relax. You're turning off the "fight-or-flight" response that occurs when you're stressed, and giving yourself more opportunities to slow down, think clearly, be thankful, and happy and healthy. It all begins one breath at a time!

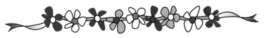

Breathing is the greatest pleasure in life – it gives life!
– Papini, 1881-1956

During your weekly 24-hour fast try to avoid criticizing anyone or anything! Fill yourself only with loving, positive thoughts, not only on your fasting and cleansing days, but everyday! Before you speak put your words to this test! "Is it good? Is it kind? Is it necessary? If not, don't speak!" – Patricia Bragg

---

Deep breathing gets more oxygen into your lungs and helps improve drainage of your lymphatic system, which removes toxins from your body. Deep breathing helps in stress relief. Slow, rhythmic, deep breathing acts as a mini meditation. Shift to slower breathing in times of tension – inhale for four counts and exhale for eight – it helps to de-stress and energize you at the same time! • doctoroz.com

Breathing Right Contributes to Happiness!

"Breathing is your body's most essential requirement for life. Without oxygen, you would only live a few minutes at most. But your breath is more than just simple movements of oxygen in and out of your lungs. It is necessary for your body functions. The air you breathe has its own energy fields or life force. This life force is in all living things on Earth. Without it, we would not be alive at all. It's this very life force, which is a combination of electric and magnetic energies and more, that is keeping our heart, lungs, kidneys, liver and all other organs pumping and functioning through electrical signals received from the brain." – *Mike Adams, Health Ranger*

A proper breathing pattern will allow you to wake up rested, keep your energy levels balanced throughout the day, decrease your waistline by improving digestion, and slow down your cellular metabolism so that you can live a long, happy life. Because your breath mirrors your mental state, you can guide your breath to become calm and slow. Calming your breath also calms the thoughts in your mind, thereby making your mind even quieter.

50

Breathing slowly and deeply can lead you into more peaceful spaces within your mind, heart and soul.

Once you develop deep breathing by practicing it every day, twice a day, it will be a very useful tool that you will always have with you. Use it whenever anything upsetting happens – before you react. Use it whenever you are aware of internal tension. Use it to help you fall asleep. Use it to deal with food cravings. Great for mild to moderate anxiety, this exercise cannot be recommended too highly. Everyone can benefit from it.

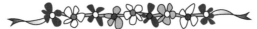

If you are honest with yourself, you will quickly discover that most of the things you truly love to do in your leisure time are not only simple, but also free and surprisingly healthy. So, instead of rushing out to see the latest film or show, why not watch the sunset? Take a walk in nature alone or with a loved one! Read a favorite book or listen to your favorite music! Relax and enjoy!

Miracles can happen every day through guidance and prayer! – Patricia Bragg

Chapter 9

Powerful Benefits of Bragg Super Power Breathing

A strong mind in a strong healthy body.

The Ancient Greek civilization, which produced some of the greatest minds the world has known, lived by the motto: *A strong mind in a strong body.* The Ancient Greeks were noted for their amazing powers of endurance, robust health and youthful longevity! All of these were the results of their systems of natural eating, deep breathing and strenuous exercise, which produced physiques that have served as the models of classical art ever since.

The classic Greeks followed 4 main health principles:

1. Full, deep, super power breathing.
2. Eating two meals of natural, healthy foods per day.
3. Exercising for complete body development.
4. Honoring supreme health, body, mind and soul.

 51

We can do the same and achieve the same results they did. We can become more vital and totally fit – enjoying every minute of being alive! The time to start is NOW – whatever your calendar years. Whether you are a teenager or a great-grandparent or somewhere in between, it is never too early or too late to start on your Supreme Road to Super Health!

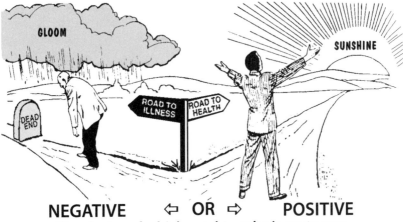

NEGATIVE ⇦ OR ⇨ POSITIVE
The choice of which road to take is up to you.

You alone decide whether to reach a dead end or live a healthy lifestyle for a long, healthy, happy, active life. – Paul C. Bragg

Super Power Breathing Promotes Healthy Body

The most important of all physical acts is correct breathing. The rhythm and depth of your breath directly affects the state of your mind and the health of your body. You can not be 100% healthy if you don't breathe deeply. Taking deeper breaths will bring more oxygen into your body and improve your energy levels! Deep breathing is not only important for living longer but also to have a good mood and keep performing at your best.

Here are benefits of deep breathing and why you should make it a part of your daily living:

✴ *Deep Breathing Detoxifies and Releases Toxins.* The body is designed to release 70% of its toxins through breathing. If you are not breathing effectively, you are not ridding your body of toxins. Then the other systems of your body must work overtime which could eventually lead to illness.

✴ *All Internal Organs are Massaged.* The movements of the diaphragm during deep breathing exercise massage the stomach, small intestine, liver and the pancreas.

✴ *Respiratory System Works Better.* Difficulties such as asthma, bronchitis and other respiratory systems and even chest pain can subside (see info on pages 79-89).

✴ *Digestive System Does Its Job.* Digestive ills (poor digestion, bloating, constipation) are helped by the internal massage of correct diaphragmatic action. When a Super Power Breath is taken, the digestive tract gets healthy exercise. Deep optimal breathing is the great body health normalizer. Oxygen, the invisible staff of life, is food for the body and helps with assimilation of foods. Oxygen burns calories and helps promote normal, healthy weight. The digestive organs receive more oxygen and operate more efficiently.

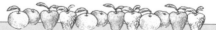

"To stop heartburn, gerd, indigestion and improve digestion, sip 1/2 tsp. organic apple cider vinegar with water before meals."
– Dr. Gabriel Cousens, M.D., author, *Conscious Eating*

Stop chewing gum – it causes stomach and digestive problems and fools the body into thinking food is coming. Chewing starts the digestive juices flowing. These powerful juices can cause trouble with your empty stomach's lining, resulting in stomach ulcers, heartburn, bloating, and gas.

✳ *Lymph System Works Better.* Increases circulation of lymphatic fluid which speeds recovery after illnesses.

✳ *Circulation System Moves!* Many people suffer from poor circulation in various parts of the body. Because they don't get sufficient oxygen to produce a steady blood circulation into their extremities, they have cold hands, feet, noses and ears. The more oxygen you get into your body, the better for your circulation and heart, and your hands and feet will be warmer! When more oxygen gets into your bloodstream, you will feel super energized and have greater super vitality to better enjoy a longer, healthier, happier life! See web: *breatheology.com*

✳ *Immune System has More Energy.* Deep Breathing creates more energy for the body to heal and detoxify. Helps tissues to regenerate and heal. Enriches your blood cells to metabolize nutrients and vitamins. Super Power Breathing is now a part of all cures. Today, in the modern hospital, pure oxygen heals when every other method of healing has failed. Even broken bones heal more quickly when the blood is purified by doing daily Super Power Breathing Exercises. Oxygen – the great invisible food for life, stimulant and purifier – builds our health resistance to infections and strengthens our weak points. It's our most vital aid in helping the body to heal itself and to stay healthy!

✳ *Cleansing Systems Works Better.* Excess fluids are eliminated through deep breathing. The stress on organs is lessened, allowing the body to cleanse naturally.

✳ *Blood Quality Improves.* When you regularly breathe oxygen correctly, you are adding millions of health-giving, oxygen-carrying red blood cells to your bloodstream, your miracle river of life. Deep Breathing removes all the carbon-dioxide and increases oxygen in the blood.

✳ *Nervous System Improves.* The brain, spinal cord and nerves receive increased oxygen. This improves the health of the whole body, since the nervous system communicates to all parts of the body. Many nervous diseases are due to oxygen starvation. Deep, diaphragmatic breathing tranquilizes jangled nerves and stimulates the brain with clear thinking and more alertness to help solve life's problems and make wise decisions (see more page 55).

✳ *Lungs are Strengthened.* When you fill your lungs with more miracle-working oxygen, you cleanse your body of toxic poisons that could do your body great health damage. As you breathe deeply the lungs become healthier and more powerful. Good insurance against respiratory problems.

✳ *Heart Grows Stronger.* Slow, deep breaths soothe and recharge the heart. Conversely, rapid, shallow breathing exhausts it through overwork and lack of sufficient oxygen for the blood. Since the heart doesn't have to work as hard to deliver oxygen to the tissues, the heart can rest a little.

✳ *Muscles Get a Workout.* When you breathe easier you move easier! Deep breathing increases flexibility, strengthens joints and supplies oxygen to brain and all cells in your body which increases the muscles in your body.

✳ *Emotionally You Feel Better.* People who deeply inhale larger amounts of oxygen are happier people. Super Power Breathing cleanses your body of psychological and physical poisons and gives you more joyful daily living and emotional well-being (see pages 48-50).

✳ *Reduces Feelings of Stress.* Deep breathing relaxes the body and releases endorphins – natural pain-killers that create natural highs – and make it easier to sleep. Deep breathing will help clear uneasy feelings out of your body.

✳ *You Become Mentally Present.* Mental observation and concentration is improved. There is greater productivity, insight, learning and better decision making.

✳ *Physical Appearance Improves.* People who get ample oxygen sleep better and have better muscle tone. Skin is healthier, firmer and more alive! Oxygen is Mother Nature's great miracle beautifier. It gives the skin a radiant glow and the hair a lustrous sheen.

You will have fewer wrinkles from improved circulation. Breathing helps create beautiful skin at any age! Good breathing techniques will also encourage good posture, which in turn helps you to look and feel younger (see posture exercise page 165). If you are overweight, the extra oxygen helps burn up excess fat more efficiently.

There are only two ways to live your life. One way is as though nothing is a miracle. The other way is as everything is a miracle! – Albert Einstein

---

Deep breathing increases flow of blood and oxygen to heart, brain and eyes.

❋ *Increases Your Spirituality.* Deep Breathing deepens your meditation and increases your intuition when you're relaxed. It helps connect you to your inner soul which helps with "self-love" and greater compassion for others.

❋ *Promotes Super Energy!* You will no longer crave artificial stimulants (caffeine, alcohol, tobacco) when sufficient oxygen is taken into your system. Oxygen is the wise stimulant that has no harmful after-effects.

Deep, Full Breathing Helps Relieve Pain

Civilized human beings with their unhealthy, self-destructive eating and living habits tend to accumulate latent poisons in their bodies. This means that the body stockpiles toxic poisons in different areas when they could not be disposed of through the body's regular avenues of elimination. These poisons are stored in veins, arteries, joints, organs, tissues, skin, etc. When they accumulate and press on nerves and tissues, there is pain. You may think this pain is new, but it's usually a *flare-up* of the old stored-up body toxins (except in cases of injury).

B-Complex, Magnesium and Deep Breathing Improves Brain Function and Soothes Nerve

55

When an emotional upset occurs, which inevitably befalls each of us, go off by yourself and take long, slow, relaxed breaths. Soon you'll find your nerves quieting down and more logical thinking will replace emotionalism. You will become master of the situation and better able to calmly resolve your problem. (Magnesium, B12, B-Complex or their injections help breathing, calm nerves and improve brain function. St. John's Wort also helps.) Read our book *Building Powerful Nerve Force & Positive Energy* for improving nerve health.

Man is the sole and absolute master of his own fate forever. What he has sown in times of ignorance, he must inevitably reap; when he attains enlightenment, it is for him to sow what he chooses and reap accordingly.
– Sir Walter Scott, Scottish Poet

Minimizing your exposure to environmental toxins (ex. using air and water purifiers, eating organic foods, etc.) while restoring oxygen balance in the body is a commonsense plan for cellular rejuvenation and disease prevention. These are simple ways to improve oxygenation in your body!

Deep Breathing Helps Respiratory Ailments

Letters and case stories give testimony to the blessed relief that Bragg Super Power Breathing has brought to thousands suffering from breathing problems such as sinusitis, bronchitis, asthma and emphysema. These suffocating diseases, characterized by chronic mucus inflammation and obstruction of the air passages, have become more prevalent today as our air becomes more polluted. (Take precaution, use air purifiers and humidifiers for home, office and your car, see page 115.) In fact, colds, flu and chronic sinus inflammation are the most common illnesses seen by doctors today (backaches are second).

Breathing Exercises Stimulate Pituitary Gland

Stimulation of the body's master gland, the pituitary, is one of the greatest benefits of Bragg Super Power Breathing Exercises. *The pituitary gland is located at the base of the brain and is the master miracle of every human act and unconscious function occurring within the heart and abdominal cavity.* It determines a person's height, length of their bones, muscle and pulse strength, mental activity and even lifespan.

The pituitary is the master gland of life and controls the functions of all other body glands. The more oxygenated blood you give the pituitary gland, the greater output of all valuable body hormones. The better the glands function, the more the entire body will rejuvenate itself to stay healthier and more youthful!

This is why the following exercises are called Super Power Breathing Exercises. Although each one is directed toward a specific part of the body, all employ the same basic, super oxygen principle. They all also stimulate the master pituitary gland and brain area with super oxygen.

Better an ounce of prevention, than a pound of cure!
Start now to breathe deeply and live fully!

Now I see the secret of making the best persons, it is to grow in the open air, live simple and eat natural foods and sleep with Mother Earth. – Walt Whitman

Improper breathing is a common cause of ill health. Changing and improving your breathing can affect you emotionally and physically. – Dr. Andrew Weil

56

Chapter 10

Preparing for
Bragg Super Power Breathing
What is Bragg Super Power Breathing?

Bragg Super Power Breathing is based upon simple, natural laws. The more oxygen you get into the body, the more carbon dioxide poison you will eliminate from the body. When oxygen replaces carbon dioxide, there will be greater purification of the blood, cells and organs of the body for improved health and a longer life!

Thousands upon thousands of lives have been saved with oxygen therapy! It is a well established scientific fact that, when all known conventional methods of healing fail, oxygen thereby is used to save lives. So, if pure oxygen can save the lives of humans who are on the brink of death, is it not logical that inhaling more oxygen deeply can prolong our lives? Or that it will free us from toxins that bring pain and distress to our physical bodies and give us a greater enjoyment of life?

57

Oxygen is the only stimulant upon which you can safely rely as a depression chaser and body builder. Bragg Super Power Breathing's main purpose is to get more life-giving oxygen into all parts of your body for health.

Bragg Super Power Breathing Exercises should not be confused with physical exercises. While this kind of breathing does produce more energy and physical and nerve strength, it has nothing to do with mere muscular development. However, it is almost impossible to have ample oxygen freely circulating in the body without beneficial effects occurring throughout. Extra benefits will be healthier muscle tone, more firmness of the skin and improved posture. Oxygen is a miracle normalizer!

The basic principle of Bragg Super Power Breathing is to fill the lungs to capacity with oxygen, then holding breath in, lean forward and drop your head below your heart. This uses the force of gravity to infuse the head's cavities with oxygenated blood, which energizes the brain and helps maintain and create new brain cells (see Salk Institute page 16).

Overcoming the Effects of Bad Breathing

The Bragg Breathing Exercises and Healthy Lifestyle work to tone and regulate your entire body to make it healthier. Most humans are victims of two bad habits: shallow breathing and incorrect posture. Both must be overcome! Muscles must be strengthened, especially the diaphragm and the abdominal muscles. Unused lung air sacs must be opened and revitalized fully with oxygen.

Perhaps you have already experienced a *stitch in the side* when you have had to run to catch a bus or plane, or while doing some unaccustomed exercise. Actually this can be a good sign, if you will profit by it. It is good to exercise to the point of getting that *stitch*. What it really means is that you have discovered a large area of unused lung cells, which have remained closed most of your life, since childhood. Now your lungs are opening to receive the fresh air you are pumping in through your efforts to breathe more deeply. The diaphragms of older people can become semi-paralyzed from non-use, but with exercise and Bragg Super Power Deep Breathing that can change!

As lung cells suffer disuse they begin to stick together and collapse in upon themselves. The sharp pain is due to the air forcing these cells apart. Continue to breathe deeply, even after you have caught the bus, plane or stopped your exercise, run, etc. The distress soon passes and your unused lung cells will soon become reactivated! You will then have made an important step forward in Bragg Super Power Breathing and achieving greater super vitality and health.

If you experience that *stitch* during the preparatory exercises which we are going to outline, you will now understand what it is caused by and not be alarmed. Just keep doing your deep breathing for more super energy!

TEST See if you are a chest breather or abdomen breather: Place right hand on chest and left hand on abdomen. As you breathe, see which hand rises more. If right hand rises more, you are a chest breather. If left hand rises more, you are an abdomen breather. – See web: www.LiveStrong.com.

Remember: "It is NEVER too late to be what you might have been!"

Fresh Air and Warmth are Necessary

Sleep in a well-ventilated (airy) room on a firm mattress. Use natural cotton percale or flannel sheets. These fabrics and silk are also preferred for bedtime wear, or wear nothing. Don't use electric blankets or heating pads, because they can disturb your body's natural currents and even be harmful to health, state scientists. If you must, only use to pre-warm, then unplug!

Be sure there's ample fresh air circulating in your room. If not, do these exercises before an open window. We want you to get full benefit of these stimulating breathing exercises and to enjoy every minute of them. If it's too cool when you get out of bed, put on something that is loose and warm. We often wear cozy sweatshirts and sweatpants.

As you start doing your exercises you will soon feel a wonderful glow of circulation coming over your entire body as you become warmer. When you feel warm enough, peel off your sweat clothes and get right down to your bare skin. Remember that you also breathe through your skin! It's an important organ of respiration – your skin and billions of pores are often called your *third lung*.

Air Baths are Health Builders

Give yourself an external as well as an internal air bath. Let your approximately two billion pores breathe in the breath of life, too. The pores of your body will welcome the contact with fresh air. They are wrapped up in clothes all day and probably at night also, unless you sleep in the nude. Daily air baths (babies love them too) do wonders for the skin. No creams can give you *"skin you love to touch"* like fresh air can! A daily private (nude) air bath also greatly enhances your skin's primary function as the main thermostatic regulator (control) of your body's temperature. This practice helps condition the skin to adjust to hot and cold weather more easily. It's a faithful thermostat when you treat it well. But if you keep your body heavily clothed and overheated all the time, your skin becomes like a hothouse plant,

---

May you live all the days of your life. – Jonathan Swift

unable to withstand drastic temperature changes. When you allow your entire body to breathe freely in the nude, your body's thermostat learns to readjust itself so that it works perfectly for you in hot and cold weather! (Also, try this powerful combination 2-3 times weekly: air bath and light skin brushing – page 197.)

Enjoy Early Morning Breathing Exercises

Upon awakening in the morning it's ideal to first do some slow body stretching exercises. Then super-charge your day with a peak supply of oxygen energy by doing 10-15 minutes of Super Power Breathing Exercises. After your exercises enjoy a glass of apple cider vinegar mixed with 1-2 tsps. raw honey (optional) in a glass of distilled water (recipe on page 144). For more information read these two books: *Apple Cider Vinegar – Miracle Health System* and *Water – The Shocking Truth* (see back pages for Bragg booklist).

The early morning hours are especially important for doing these breathing exercises, especially if a city dweller, because air is less polluted then. These exercises will jump start your day with super energy that will carry you through whatever challenges may arise. You will become more confident, stronger and healthier.

Think of this health-building period with pleasant anticipation. It's a time to build your vitality, energy, strength and all the good things that come to a healthy body. Go into it with dedicated self-responsibility and enthusiasm. Your faithful efforts will bring super results!

Practice Bragg Posture Exercises Every Day

Correct posture (see pages 161-166) allows the chest to expand so the lungs can be filled with air. The lungs inflate with air like millions of tiny balloons. Suction is created below by the action of the diaphragm and above by the auxiliary muscles of the chest and abdomen. This suction fills your lungs with air. The lungs themselves are passive and cannot breathe independently. The lungs wait patiently to be refilled with air. So now make it a habit to breathe deeply to help keep your lungs and body healthy.

Remember, the lungs are attached to the rib cage walls by pleural membranes. If the sternum, or breastbone, is carried high and the bony rib cage expanded, the lungs are held up with good posture so they can be easily filled with air. The uplifted diaphragm, in turn, tends to draw into position any sagging or prolapsed stomach organs.

As with deep breathing, most young children exhibit good posture naturally, only to lose both as they mature! To make matters worse, most occupations today (from assembly line to desk jobs) have a tendency to pull us down from an erect, good posture position. The result is that many people carry themselves like a collapsed accordion, shoulders sagging, chest deflated, which puts their heart, organs and breathing apparatus in a tight viselike grip!

⬚1⬚ See posture exercise (page 165) to help counteract this unhealthy and energy-sapping poor posture. Now stand with feet 10" apart and stretch hands high overhead, at the same time rising high on toes. See how high you can lift up your chest while drawing in abdominal muscles. Stretch up and up, as if trying to touch the ceiling. *Now drop arms. Relax and repeat this exercise 10 times.* Do not try to do any special breathing. Just breathe naturally, or what is natural for you at the time.

This stretching exercise is designed to strengthen the muscles which control the erect posture of the body. Stretching is one of the greatest tools for building health. It is the universal exercise of the animal kingdom. Wild animals are beautiful examples of instinctual natural living. Also, your pets (cats, dogs, birds, etc.) all wisely stretch daily. *When you sit awhile, stand up and do some stretching exercises!*

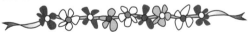

He who can't find time for exercise will have time for illness. – Lord Derby

---

A healthy body is a guest-chamber for the soul; a sick body is a prison.
– Francis Bacon, 1st Viscount of St Alban and English philosopher

---

As often as possible make yourself smile and laugh; it opens the blood vessels in the back of your head to physically lift your mood. Choose to be happy in spite of circumstances. You can make yourself happy, it's your inner Nerve Force and attitude that sparkles from within.

Stomach Muscles Need These Exercises

Most people allow their stomach muscles to be lazy, flabby and unhealthy. Carrying excess belly fat around the waistline can impair lung function. Abdominal obesity is defined as having a waistline of greater than 35" for women and 40" for men. French researchers think belly fat may impair the way the diaphragm and chest function. A good time to strengthen, tone and control these natural girdle muscles is to practice these two exercises every morning before getting out of bed. Remember your waistline is your lifeline!

2 Lying on your back – fix your eyes and attention on your stomach. Now start moving your stomach muscles upwards, then force them downwards. Wiggle your insides, in one direction, then another, then from side to side, letting your hands help at first. When you discover you can control your stomach muscles in one movement, then practice the other movements. Do daily for results!

Thinking about and using these stomach muscles is just the beginning. The goal of these exercises is the ability to control the abdominal muscles in the same way you do those of the legs and arms. Your stomach muscles must do your bidding if you want to develop a useful diaphragm. After you have obtained some control over your stomach muscles while lying on your back in bed, *begin doing the same movements while standing upright.* You can accomplish much more with your muscles in this upright position.

3 Standing upright, with hands hanging relaxed at sides, draw in and up the stomach muscles until it looks like a deep valley, as though everything inside was moving up in the chest cavity. Then push your muscles out until you see your protruding belly. Now suck the muscles in, then push out. Now wiggle them up and down, and last pull in, tighten, firm and stretch up your midsection and spine. Repeat several times. This is called *Nauli Kriya.*

Your waistline is your health-line, dateline, youth-line and lifeline!
– Patricia Bragg

Man is fully responsible for his nature and his choices. – Jean-Paul Sartre

When you acquire this control over the abdomen and surrounding muscles, you will discover many benefits. Abdominal exercises strengthen the body and result in a straight, aligned spine. With a strong mid-section, the body can stand tall. Another reward is it helps you establish a more normal bowel rhythm. Usually soon after arising and within an hour after each meal there should be a bowel movement. (See simple exercise bottom of page 70.)

Diaphragm Exercise – Most Important Muscle

When exercising your abdominal muscles, you will also be exercising your diaphragm, especially in the upward and downward pushing movements. Here is a special exercise for your diaphragm: *locate your diaphragm* by placing one hand at your waistline, then with the other hand hold the palm upward in front of your mouth. Now blow imaginary dust from the palm. Where you feel a strong muscular contraction when blowing, that's the location of **your diaphragm, the most important muscle you use when doing Bragg Super Power Breathing.**

4 Walk around your room on bare tiptoes, with your hands stretching up, reaching high over your head. Raise your diaphragm as high as your strength will allow, still breathing deeply. Feel it stretch your chest and stomach muscles as you breathe deeply. Now bend over, drop head below heart, arms towards floor, then circle your arms in front of chest, compressing out every bit of toxic, carbon dioxide-laden air. Do this often, as it's a super lung cleanser and health builder.

It's a great habit to suck the oxygen-bearing fresh air deeply and slowly into your lungs. If you feel a little dizzy with the sudden oxygen stimulation, stop for a moment, then continue. *Begin by doing this diaphragm stretch – deep breathing exercise 5 times, gradually increasing to 10.* When you are able to do this exercise with ease, you are ready to start your Bragg Super Power Breathing Program (starts on page 67).

Exercise is the best natural anti-anxiety agent available. It reduces tension as it relieves aggression and frustration, aids concentration and mental focus while curbing the appetite and improving sleep.

Singing – Breathing Exercise

What is more elemental to singing than the breathing in and out of pure air into your hard-working lungs? Projecting sound and sustaining a note is hallmark of strong breathing muscles just as a lean, firm body is the sign of healthy, fit living. With singing, *(also whistling)* just as in breathing, the diaphragm and abdomen take lead roles and this exercise will help you master their use.

While standing up straight, feet 12" apart, place your left and right hand fingers on bottom ribs with thumbs gently probing below bottom rib. Now slowly draw in a full, deep diaphragmatic breath while feeling 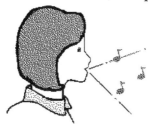 your abdominal movements with all fingers. Hold your breath for five seconds, now slowly exhale . . . but don't just "breathe out," instead, you should "sing out" the air. So, as you slowly let your breath out, softly sing a sustained note, as in "aa-hhh" or "oo-hhh." Note the abdominal movements with your **64** fingers again. Repeat exercise 3 to 5 times. This helps you extend your control over the flow of sound and breath and helps you master your miracle breathing machinery.

Candle – Breathing Exercise

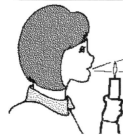 In this version of the singing exercise, instead of holding your sides you hold a candle in front of your mouth. Again, slowly sing out your breath as evenly as possible – and thus exercise mastery of your breathing by controlling the candle flame.

Nature cannot be hastened. The bloom of a flower opens in its own proper time. – Paul Bruton

---

Diaphragmatic breathing is beneficial – it enhances circulatory function and relaxes muscles of ribs, chest and stomach. – Susan Smith Jones, Ph.D.

Little deeds of kindness, little words of love and thanks, help to make earth happy, like the Heaven above. – Julia A. F. Carney

Arm Pumping – Breathing Exercise

Stretching up spine, stand tall, legs relaxed with feet 12" apart. Drop arms down at sides. Now gradually pump arms up and down bird-style, breathing in through your mouth until your arms are up above your head. Grasp hands, stretch up, hold breath for five seconds. Now slowly breathe out as you bend down, relaxed, dropping arms and head below your heart. Repeat twice.

Controlled Deep Breathing For Super Oxygen

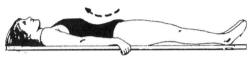

[1] Enjoy this exercise before getting up in the morning and then repeat often during your day. It's also relaxing just before sleep. Count to yourself as you gently exhale and slowly inhale (vary breathing through the mouth and the nose). When you become more adept, then increase the count.

It's challenging to have breathing contests with your mate, family and friends to see who can take the deepest, slowest, longest breaths! This exercise will strengthen your lungs, chest and all muscles around your mid-waist. It also improves lung capacity and super breathing power as it gives you a firmer, trimmer waistline. This will help you learn to breathe in and out with control, varying breathing through the mouth and nose! When on walks pay attention to how long it takes to inhale and exhale. Ideally exhaling should be longer.

65

Diaphragmatic Panting Breathing Exercise: Super Oxygenator For Super Healthy Living

[2] Raise your arms so that your ribs are separated. Rather than breathe as you normally would, pant while breathing. Pant until your diaphragm is tired. Your exhale panting should take about twice as long as your inhale panting. For example, if your inhale lasts for a count of 6, try to make your exhale last to 12. Do this exercise daily, especially before retiring. This helps re-oxygenate your entire body and remove the toxins from your system so you can enjoy a peaceful, restful and recharging sleep.

One-Breath Meditation Works Miracles

3 ATP (adenosine triphosphate) is a naturally occurring by-product of breathing that regulates physical action, thought and feeling. Dips in ATP levels can cause fatigue, aches and pains. The one-breath meditation exercise helps reverse the falling levels of important needed ATP.

1. *Sit in a comfortable chair and straighten up your spine, keeping shoulders back and relaxed.*

2. *Now inhale slowly and deeply, clear your mind completely. Relax shoulders and back. Imagine yourself in a secret garden, deeply drawing in peace and vitality from the oxygen rich air.*

3. *Hold your breath for a moment, then exhale slowly and fully, releasing all the tension from all your muscles and body.*

Use this one minute refresher at home, work and throughout the day as needed to refresh, restore and recharge your body, mind and soul – it works miracles!

Breathing Exercises During Pregnancy and Childbirth Benefit Mother and Baby

In natural childbirth classes (waterbirth, birthing chair, etc.) parents are taught certain breathing techniques, such as Lamaze or Bradley, to help make childbirth easier and more comfortable. Mothers who practice the Bragg Super Breathing throughout their pregnancies have stronger muscles. This enhances their ability to make use of other breathing techniques and helps make the birthing process easier: ensuring the mother and baby will have a healthier, happier, birthing experience. The primary benefits for the mother are a shortened recovery time and the ability to fully participate in the joyful process of her child's birth. For the baby, the primary benefit comes from the well-oxygenated blood the mother had been providing for the nine months she carried the child in her womb. This oxygen helps prevent birth defects and helps ensure that the baby is born healthier and ready for a healthy, long life!

Man's precious breath is the gift of life from God.
With the care and nurturing of this life gift, all health and wisdom is ours.

Chapter 11

Bragg Super Power Breathing Exercises

Faithfulness counts towards super health.

The basic principle of Bragg Super Power Breathing is to fill the lungs to capacity with oxygen, then hold breath in, leaning forward, drop your head below your heart. This uses the force of gravity to infuse the head's cavities with oxygenated blood, which energizes the brain and helps maintain and create new brain cells (see page 16).

Every person who is interested in Super Health should take time each morning to do these Super Power Breathing Exercises. Take your present physical condition into consideration when you start on this program. Go slowly at first. Large parts of your lungs have probably been dormant for some time! It will take time to gradually open up these areas. Daily exercises will bring miracle results.

Make these exercises a daily habit, as much a part of your life as dressing, brushing your teeth and eating. The wonderful results obtained from faithfully following these breathing exercises and lifestyle will repay you abundantly with more health, energy, peace and longevity!

67

Many people go through their life committing partial suicide. They destroy their health, youth, talents, energies and creative qualities. Indeed, to learn how to be good to oneself is often harder than to learn how to be good to others.
– Joshua Liebman, Ph.D., author "Peace of Mind"

Nature, time and patience are the 3 greatest physicians. – Wise Irish Proverb

---

Accuse not nature, she hath done her part; now do thine!
– John Milton, author "Paradise Lost"

Breathing only in the upper chest avoids the strong creative energies of the abdomen and sexual organs. Breathing only in the abdomen avoids the powerfully creative energies of the heart and throat. – Michael G. White

Exercise 1 – The Cleansing Breath

This is your Basic Super Power Breathing Exercise.
All Super Power Breathing Exercises begin this way. Stand erect, feet about 15 to 18 inches apart, hands and arms relaxed at your sides (figure a). Raise your hands overhead (figure b). Now bend forward as far as possible – keeping your knees slightly bent and relaxed – exhaling at the same time through your mouth. Compress your chest and push upward with your diaphragm and abdominal muscles to expel all the stale air out of your lungs (figure c).

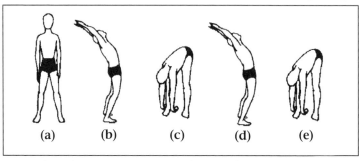

(a)   (b)   (c)   (d)   (e)

Now slowly inhale air through nose and mouth, pushing air downward with diaphragm and expanding your chest at its front and sides. Continue to draw in air to the full capacity of your lungs as you return to a standing position, while bringing your arms upward in a half-circle to the overhead position (figure d).

To complete the Cleansing Breath Exercise: As your hands reach the overhead position, tighten your diaphragm and hold your breath for four or five seconds (mentally counting, *one thousand one, one thousand two,* etc.) while pulling your abdominal muscles back as if to pin your stomach to your backbone. Then exhale completely while bending forward, as in figure c & e. Now inhale as you return up as figure b and repeat exercise. Do this Cleansing Breath Exercise five times.

The quality of breath should be deep, graceful, easy and efficient.
– Kenneth Cohen

Idleness of mind and body is the slow burial of a living man. – Jeremy Taylor

It's never too late to get into shape, but it does take daily perseverance.
– Dr. Thomas K. Cureton – Physical Fitness Pioneer, University of Illinois

Exercise 2 – The Super Power Brain Breath

Start by exhaling and inhaling as in Exercise 1. When your hands reach the overhead position, hold your breath (hold nose closed if necessary) and bend forward from the waist, knees bent, dropping your head below your heart, downward as far as possible. Continue to hold your breath to the count of 10 (mentally counting, *One thousand one, one thousand two,* etc.). This exercise allows the richly oxygenated blood to suffuse the pituitary gland on its way to reaching, refreshing and recharging every part of your brain for sharper thinking (work, school, etc.). This power breathing also helps cleanse the skull cavities (important and vital sinuses, ears, nose, eyes and mouth).

While holding your breath, now return to a standing position. Then bend forward, exhaling vigorously through the mouth. Slowly inhale as you return to starting standing position. Do this exercise five times at the beginning, gradually increasing to 10 repetitions.

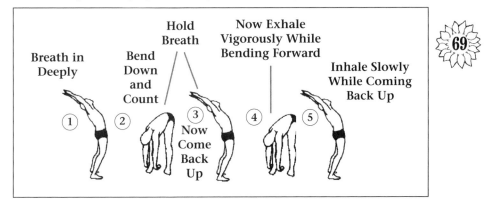

69

NOTE: In these exercises, you may not be able to hold your breath for the full count at first. If you begin to feel dizzy, exhale and return to the standing position, dropping your arms to your sides and relax for a few minutes before continuing the exercise. You will gradually build your oxygen tolerance and be able to do the full count.

Health and intellect are two blessings of life. – Menander

Nothing transforms as much as changing from a negative to a positive attitude!

You are never too old to set another goal or to dream a new dream. – C.S. Lewis

Exercise 3 – The Super-Kidney Breath

Locate your kidneys (lower back, just below the end of your rib cage near the waistline). Get the *feel* of them by placing your palms over this area, fingers and thumbs pointed downward. Use this position during the breath-holding part.

Exhale and inhale like the beginning of Exercise 1. As your hands reach the overhead position, tighten your diaphragm and pin your stomach to your backbone with your abdominal muscles, while holding your breath. Then firmly place your palms, with light pressure, over your kidneys, relax knees and bend backward for a silent count of 10. Still holding your breath, return to standing position. Then bend forward while exhaling vigorously through the mouth. (Use same precautions as in Exercise 2.) Slowly inhale as you return to the starting position. Do this exercise five times at the start, gradually increasing to 10.

Exercise 4 – For Easier Flowing Bowels

Do this exercise in the bathroom soon after rising each morning, and several times within an hour after eating. If you make this a habit, you will soon find you will have a bowel movement upon arising and an hour after eating. Taking a psyllium husk veg. cap after dinner works great!

Exhale and inhale as beginning Exercise 1. Now, holding breath, clasp hands in front and slowly lower yourself into relaxed squatting position while still holding your breath. Then strain for bowel movement for several seconds. Return to standing position exhaling and inhaling as in previous exercises. Note: Squatting is a natural way to have easy bowel movements. Children squat naturally. It opens up the anal area more directly. Putting feet up on a wastebasket or footstool when on the toilet gives the same effect. Also stretch arms up above head so transverse colon will empty easier.

ELIMINATE THE "DRIBBLES" EXERCISE: To keep bladder and sphincter muscles tight and toned, urinate – stop – urinate – stop, 4 times, twice daily when voiding, especially after age of 40. This simple exercise works wonders for both men and women!

Exercise 5 – Filling the Lungs

This exercise is designed to get oxygen into the little-used air sacs at the bottom (apex) of the lungs, down near your waistline. Exhale and inhale as at the start of Exercise 1. But instead of returning the arms to the overhead position, relax them at your sides and bring your feet together, toes and heels touching. While holding your breath, bend to the right and reach toward the floor with the fingers of your right hand, at the same time bringing the left hand up to touch under the left armpit. Hold this position for a silent count of 10. Return to starting position and exhale and inhale as before. Now repeat the breath-holding position on your left side. Reach toward floor with left hand while placing right hand under right armpit for a count of 10. Repeat this exercise 5 to 10 times, alternating sides.

Exercise 6 – The Super Power Liver Cleansing Breath

Exhale and inhale as at the beginning of Exercise 1. Now bring feet together and clasp your fingers overhead, palms upward. Keep legs stiff from the hips down. Now holding a full breath, bend slowly to right side, then the left side, with as much stretch as possible. Now after doing left and right side stretches, return to starting position, but with feet apart. Next exhale with the usual forward bend, forcing all the old air out and then breathe in as you come up. Do 5 sets, gradually increasing to 10 repetitions of this liver cleansing exercise that promotes cleansing and circulation.

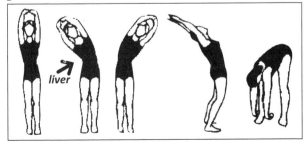

Modern society lives in an unhealthy way that produces many over-worked livers. When we overeat, eat junk foods, and are exposed to environmental pollutants and stress, the liver becomes overworked and overloaded! – GlobalHealing.com

Exercise 7 – Heart Strengthener

The purpose of this exercise is to expand the aorta, the main trunk of the arterial system which carries the blood from the heart after it has been oxygenated by Super Power Breathing. This exercise stimulates the circulation of blood in the heart, as well as the entire body, cardiovascular system, etc. It also helps recharge and increase the power of the respiratory system. This exercise also helps give relief to those who suffer from the feelings of suffocation and apprehension caused by asthma, angina pectoris, etc. (See Healthy Heart Habits page 174. Live a healthy lifestyle, plus drink eight glasses of distilled water daily.)

This exercise starts with exhaling and inhaling as in the beginning of Exercise 1 (page 68), except that the arms are held forward at shoulder height (not overhead). When you return to the standing position, hold your breath – clasp your nose tightly with thumb and index finger so that no air escapes. Then pretend you are blowing your nose. You should feel some air pressure in your ears.

Now, with knees bent, bend over from the waist and gently bring your head down below your heart and midriff. Continue to hold your breath for a silent count of 10.

Return to the starting position and exhale and inhale in the usual Bragg Super Power Breathing manner (see page 68). Repeat this exercise five times, gradually increasing to 10 repetitions.

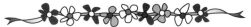

Coronary heart disease is due to a lack of oxygen received by the heart.
– Dr. Dean Ornish, author of "Stress, Diet and Your Heart"

Symptoms of heart failure reflect the diminished blood flow to all organs in the body, especially the lungs, kidneys, and liver. Such symptoms include shortness of breath, difficulty breathing when lying down and swelling in lower extremities or lower back. Take CoQ10 for a healthier heart. – LifeExtension.com

---

Always do what is right – despite any public opinions.

Cultivate the Habit of Deep Breathing: Diaphragmatic Breathing promotes a more relaxed state and makes the heart's job easier. Take a long, slow, deep breath right now! Visualize the air filling the lower part of your lungs. Do this for three minutes every hour during the day and notice the improvement.

Chapter 12

Breathing Exercises to Enjoy For More Super Energy

The Bragg Super Power Breathing exercises are powerful for super health! Here are ways to add more variety for your enjoyment. Make some or all of these exercises a part of your daily health routine to give you more super vitality, health, creativity and fitness in your life.

Posture Breathing Exercise

The following activity is designed to correct bad posture habits, which are among the greatest impediments to proper breathing. Practice this activity several times a day at the job and at home. It will bring relief to your tired shoulders, spine and eyes, making you more alert and energized.

While you're sitting relaxed in a chair, then let your chin rest on your upper chest as you slowly lean forward, slowly exhaling. With eyes closed continue leaning until hands and elbows rest comfortably on your upper legs. After slowly exhaling in this position, sit upright quickly while sniffing in a full breath of fresh air through the nose. As you do this let your eyes open wide and then hold your full breath for 10 seconds (if necessary, first begin with holding for 5 second counts).

Take special note of how the sudden inhalation works to force your posture to healthy alignment as you sit up straight. After holding the inhaled breath, slowly release air through the mouth. Then close your eyes, lean forward and then repeat the exercise two more times.

Super Power Breathing for Fresh, New Air

Because the majority of people don't use their full lungs' capacity, the following exercise is designed to get new air into the forgotten, unused regions of the lungs. Practice moderately at first, but with greater frequency as your lungs will soon become healthier and stronger!

73

Comfortably sit or stand and now inhale slowly through the nose a complete, deep diaphragmatic breath. As you do this let your head be comfortably lifted backwards until it has come to rest as far back as it can without strain. After holding this position and your breath for 3 to 5 seconds, slowly exhale through closed teeth as your head moves forward to the starting position. As you exhale (there should be a hissing noise as the air is forced between the teeth) concentrate on expelling all of the old air out of your lungs. Repeat this exercise several times. It's particularly suitable to pre-aerobic warm-ups because it will prepare the lungs for super oxygenation.

Rejuvenation Breathing Exercise

When areas of the lungs have remained unused, the pathways can become narrowed or even closed. This breathing exercise helps rejuvenate the lungs by opening up the passageways to the lungs' neglected areas! Do this activity moderately and gently at first. But as your lungs become healthier and stronger, increase the frequency and enjoy the force of your breathing exertion.

While standing, take in a deep, full diaphragmatic breath and lift your chin up slightly. Once you have taken in the full breath, hold it in and stand still. Then raise your bent arms chest high and with closed fists gently pound your upper chest area (still holding your breath) in gorilla style. Also pound your rib areas and the lower lung region. Do this for as long as you can comfortably hold your breath. As you exhale, knees relaxed, bend head down below heart and exhale as much old air as possible from your lungs. Repeat this exercise several times.

With a full breath swelling your lungs, this gentle pounding (patting) exercise opens up those passageways that haven't carried air for a long time. The more passages you have available to move air through your lungs and into your blood, the more energy and vitality and the better health and fitness you will experience.

To desire to be healthy is an important part of being healthy.
– Seneca, Roman Philosopher, 65 A.D.

Exercise to Increase Lungs' Air Space

This breathing exercise helps you make use of your lungs' maximum breathing capacity in a comfortable and gentle manner. Practice several times a day to enjoy more energy and fitness on the job and at home.

While standing, knees relaxed, bend over and exhale completely all the old stale air. You can help your lungs expel (push out) the air by pulling in your belly muscles, forcing your stomach inwards towards your spine. Now stand straight, slowly inhale, filling your lungs to full capacity and hold your breath for 20 seconds (if 20 seconds is not possible, set a challenging, non-painful goal). As you count, slowly stretch your arms up over your head. This will stretch your lungs, maximizing their air space. When you have completed your breath holding pattern, relax and bend down and exhale air slowly. Do this 2 or 3 more times and increase as desired.

Exercise for A Flexible, Youthful Rib Cage

75

As with the preceding exercise, this maximizes the body's spatial capacity for breathing. The previous exercise works on increasing the lungs' air holding capacity. This exercise works on the space your rib cage can make available for your lungs to expand.

While standing, exhale completely with arms at your sides. Slowly inhale, filling your lungs to capacity and hold your breath for 20 seconds. As you count place your palms on your hips with your thumbs forward and your pinkie fingers touching each other at your lower spine.

Now pull elbows backward far as possible while holding your breath. Then exhale slowly moving arms down to sides. Repeat 2 or 3 times. This exercise helps keep the rib area flexible, so to maximize your air lung space.

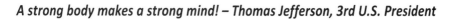

A strong body makes a strong mind! – Thomas Jefferson, 3rd U.S. President

 We must always change, renew, rejuvenate ourselves; otherwise, we harden. – Johann Wolfgang von Goethe

Exercise To Maximize Chest Area

This exercise will also help you maximize the available chest and rib cage area for your lungs to expand and take in more air. Practice several times daily along with the other air capacity increasing exercises.

Starting position – stand with your arms at sides, inhale deeply through the nose, then while holding your breath for 5 seconds, extend arms forward, now clasp hands together and stretch hands up, high above your head, exhaling quickly and fully through your mouth. Naturally your upper chest will move upward with this high up stretch. Now return to starting position and repeat 2 or 3 times.

Breathing Exercise for Lower Lungs

The lungs' lower regions are the most distant from your windpipe, and the most dependent on the breathing activity of the diaphragm. As a result, the lungs' lower regions are the most likely areas to suffer disuse. This important exercise is designed to bring more air to these under-used areas of the lungs.

76

While lying on the floor on an 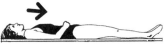 exercise/yoga mat, concentrate on your lower lungs. Put tip of index finger just below your belly button and consider this spot the center of your lower lungs. Slowly inhale through the nose a full and total breath, concentrating on filling the lung area beneath your finger first. With practice you will soon find that you can easily target your breathing in this way. As you inhale fill your lower lungs first (beneath finger), moving to your familiar upper lungs last.

After a few days of practice your skill level in this exercise will noticeably increase and you will find it easy to aim your breathing to different regions of your lungs. Once you have this ability, practice this exercise while standing or lying down, at home or at work. You will find that it is both soothing and invigorating, and suitable both for before sleep and for energy when tired.

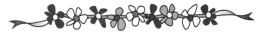

Nerve Force contains much of its power in the breath. – Yoga Teachings

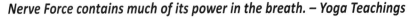

Deep, Slow Breathing
Promotes Relaxed, Peaceful Sleep

Millions worldwide suffer from insomnia – bad sleep and bad sleeping habits. Preparing sensibly for a good night's rest with a ventilated room and firm mattress are some of the easiest ways to improve your ability to sleep well (for more tips see pages 92-94). The following deep breathing exercise relaxes the body and reduces mental stress to prepare for a peaceful, recharging sleep so vital to your health and well-being!

Lie in bed on your back with hands at your sides, palms down. Close your eyes and quiet your mind as you slowly inhale through your nose to fill your lower lungs first. As you inhale, raise your arms in a slow circling motion up over your head. Aim to complete your inhalation just as your two thumbs touch each other, with arms then resting behind your head. Hold this breath for 10-15 seconds. Exhale slowly through mouth as you reverse your arm circling motion, bringing arms back to starting position at sides. Repeat this exercise several times or until relaxed and drowsy.

Another breathing technique you may try, when you first get into bed: 1) Take a deep breath. 2) Breathe in through your nose and visualize the air moving down to your stomach. 3) As you breathe in again silently count to four. 4) Purse your lips as you exhale slowly. 5) This time count silently to eight. 6) Repeat this process 6-10 times.

The results of this breathing technique are immediate. You will feel your shoulders and arms relaxing. Your chest will feel less constricted and you will feel less stress and tension! The goal is to relax your mind and let your body unwind and surrender to peaceful sleep.

For Insomnia and Nervous Tension use these Herbs:

Chamomile oil: put in bath water (5-6 drops) to soothe nerves, dilute to 2% to make an excellent massage oil. **Chamomile tea:** 2-3 times daily.

Passion Flower: for insomnia due to worry, overwork or nervous exhaustion. Excellent sedative with no side effects. Drink tea three times a day.

Valerian: for insomnia or if having hard time falling asleep helps reduce night wakings with no negative effects. Drink Valerian tea as needed.

Fast Help for Panicky, Stressful Moments

Stress and fear tighten the entire body, especially the breathing muscles. Learn to relax and loosen the tightened muscles and panic and tensions will melt away.

These simple-to-do exercises will bring fast relief:

- Concentrate breathing in deeply and slowly through mouth, then slowly blow out all stress and tension.
- Wait! Don't breathe for a few seconds. While breath is out, force stomach muscles in and out four times.
- Slow shoulder rolls to ears – then roll shoulders back, down and around, then reverse rolls. Do five times.

You will soon be more relaxed and peaceful.

For a nervous stomach, do this finger acupressure:

Firmly press, massage skin between thumb and forefinger. This helps for car and plane sickness and a nervous stomach. Life is a journey of choices. Relax, be healthy, happy, peaceful and enjoy your healthy lifestyle. Count all of your blessings!

78

Try these Ten Great No-Calorie Stress Busters:

1. Turn on your favorite music and dance.
2. Enroll in a yoga class, or take tai chi, Qigong, Pilates or enjoy a stretching class.
3. Call a good friend and have some laughs.
4. Read inspiring Bragg books and health magazines.
5. Take hot herbal bubble bath or vinegar ($\frac{1}{2}$ cup) bath.
6. Go to the gym or take a brisk fresh air health walk.
7. Get a massage – best at your home when possible.
8. Write and release your feelings in your daily journal.
9. Watch an inspiring movie, comedy or travelogue.
10. Close your eyes, relax, do 'yoga breathing' – breathe in slowly through nose, letting air fill lungs completely down to the diaphragm. Hold in briefly, then exhale through the mouth slowly. See: *HealthAndYoga.com.*

Breath is the spirit of life, the concentrated power or essence of physical being.
– Dr. Andrew Weil

Chapter 13

Common Respiratory Ailments & Diseases

Breathing difficulties can come on suddenly or be a warning of a disease in the body! Breathing problems include pain, discomfort or any difficulty that interferes with the normal, natural cycle of easily inhaling and exhaling air. Respiratory diseases are becoming more common worldwide, particularly in industrialized countries like the U.S. and China. Air pollution, cigarette smoke and congested living conditions are the main problems.

Here is a list of some common breathing ailments:

- *Asthma:* A condition where airways are constricted, making breathing difficult. See pages: 81-84 for more health info on prevention and treatment of Asthma.

- *Bronchitis:* Inflammation of bronchial tubes, the airways that carry air to your lungs. It causes a cough that often brings up mucus, as well as shortness of breath, wheezing and chest tightness. See pages 85-86 for more info.

79

- *Chronic Obstructive Pulmonary Disease (COPD):* Progressive disease that makes it hard to breathe. Can cause coughing that produces large amounts of mucus, wheezing, shortness of breath and chest tightness. Cigarette smoking is the leading cause of COPD. Long term exposure to other lung irritants – air pollution, chemical fumes or dust also may contribute to COPD. See pages 87-88 for more info.

- *Dyspnea:* Shortness of Breath – feeling like you cannot get enough air. You may experience shortness of breath just once or have recurring episodes. Very strenuous exercise, extreme temperatures, obesity and high altitude can cause Dyspnea in a healthy person. Besides these, shortness of breath is likely a sign of a medical problem. **If you have unexplained shortness of breath, see a doctor as soon as possible!**

ALPHA-1 ANTITRYPSIN DEFICIENCY: An inherited disorder that may cause serious lung disease. The body does not make enough alpha-1 antitrypsin: a protein in the blood that protects lungs from inflammation caused by infection and inhaled irritants such as tobacco smoke, etc. Most common signs and symptoms caused by Alpha-1 are shortness of breath, wheezing, chronic bronchitis, chest cold, and allergies.

- **Emphysema:** Chronic lung disease, often caused by exposure to toxic chemicals or long-term exposure to tobacco smoke. Emphysema gradually damages the air sacs in the lungs, making you progressively shorter of breath. Symptoms are shortness of breath on exertion and hyperventilation (see info on COPD page 87-88).

- **Hyperventilation:** Rapid or deep breathing that can occur with anxiety or panic. *Treatment:* The goal is to raise carbon dioxide level in your blood, which helps end your symptoms. Do this old-fashioned remedy – breathe into a paper bag for 3 minutes. It helps to restore carbon dioxide/oxygen levels in the lungs.

- **Pneumonia:** Common lung infections caused by bacteria, virus, fungi or diet. Symptoms can vary from mild to severe. *Prevention:* Frequently wash hands as flu can lead to pneumonia. Live The Bragg Healthy Lifestyle including a healthy diet (see page 122) and get ample sleep. *Treatment:* Depends on cause of pneumonia, how severe symptoms are and your age and overall health. If you suspect you have pneumonia, see your doctor!

- **Respiratory Distress Syndrome (RDS):** condition where body is not receiving enough oxygen from the lungs. Injuries, accidents, infections or other conditions cause fluid to accumulate in air sacs. Then, fluid and proteins leak out from capillaries into alveoli, making whole lungs stiff. This prevents lungs from working properly. They cannot fill up with air in a normal way, neither can they get rid of carbon dioxide effectively. The signs for Respiratory Distress are: dizziness, shortness of breath, fatigue and low blood pressure. *Treatment:* patients are placed in ICU and put on air ventilator. The No. 1 priority is to raise your blood oxygen levels.

- **Sleep Apnea:** Common respiratory disorder that causes you to stop breathing briefly while you sleep. Sleep apnea can be treated. For more info see pages 98-100.

The average human inhales 3,000 gallons of air daily.
Unfortunately millions breathe contaminated, toxic and
sick air in homes, offices, work places, cities, and airplanes, etc.

Gently forced into action, most lungs will slowly rebuild themselves.

Create the kind of self you will be happy to live with all your life.
– Foster C. McClellan

Prevention Methods for Breathing Problems:

- Avoid all tobacco smoke, smog, toxic vapors, etc.
- Exercise regularly – brisk healthy walking is great fun
- Avoid pollens, dust, molds, and other allergens
- Live The Bragg Healthy Lifestyle including faithfully maintaining a healthy diet and normal healthy weight
- Wash hands with perfume-free soap frequently
- Wear a mask when working around dust and chemicals.

Millions of Americans Suffer with Asthma

Today 25 million Americans suffer from asthma, 7% are under the age of 18. Asthma accounts for almost 2 million emergency room visits and around 13 million doctor visits a year. It's one of the great maladies of our polluted, poisoned age, costing tens of billions yearly. Four thousand Americans die from asthma yearly.

Even in hospital emergency rooms with all of the modern technology and pharmacological medicine they offer, more people are dying of asthma.

Asthma is a reversible obstructive lung disease, caused by increased reaction of the airways to various stimuli. It is a chronic inflammatory condition with serious acute exacerbations. Asthma can be a life-threatening disease if not managed! Daily control is vital to living an active, productive, healthy life towards eliminating asthma.

Asthma breathing problems usually happen in short "episodes" or "attacks," but the inflammation underlying asthma is continuous. An asthma attack occurs when muscles surrounding the airway contract, narrowing air passages that are chronically swollen and inflamed. During an attack, the mucus fills the airway like a plug. When the victim breathes in, the air slides around the mucus obstructions. When the victim tries to exhale, the mucus plugs the airway, stopping the flow of air out of the lungs. Some triggers for asthma attacks are: tobacco smoke, vapors, dust, air pollution, mites, cockroach allergen, pets, mold, smoke from burning wood, sinus infections, food allergies (milk etc. see pages 37-38), burning incense, high humidity.

Asthma and Toxic Allergy Triggers

Those with asthma should be wise and cautious of the triggers that cause attacks. Some triggers are food additives, aspirin, MSG and sulfites. In your home mold grows on shower curtains, bathtubs, tiles, etc. Dust mites' favorite areas are blankets, pillows, carpets and stuffed toys. Asthma can be triggered by smoke from the burning end of a cigarette or second hand smoke. Please don't smoke or allow others to smoke in your home! Cockroach body parts and droppings may trigger asthma attacks. The dander of cats and dogs are triggers. Nitrogen Dioxide gas can irritate eyes, nose, throat and may cause shortness of breath. This gas comes from appliances that burn gas, wood and kerosene, such as BBQ's, fireplaces and car exhaust. Chemical irritants and fragrances (buy only odor-free) can also be triggers! These are found in soaps, detergents, fabric softeners, cleaners, perfumes, aftershaves, colognes, deodorants, hairsprays, mothballs, candles and air fresheners.

Gardenburger Creator Thanks Bragg Books
Cured His Asthma in a Month

82

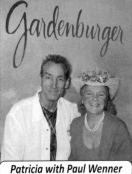

Paul Wenner, the *Gardenburger* Creator, says his early years as a youth with asthma were so bad he would stand at the window praying to breathe through the night and stay alive! A miracle happened when as a teenager he read Bragg Books on Fasting, Breathing, and Healthy Lifestyle and his years of asthma were cured in only one month! Paul became so inspired he wanted to be a Health Crusader like Paul Bragg and daughter Patricia – and Paul Wenner has! *Gardenburgers are sold worldwide. www.gardenburger.com*

Patricia with Paul Wenner

After years of asthma, in a month I could breathe normally for first time in my life.
It was a miracle! I thank Paul Bragg and Patricia for Bragg Fasting and Breathing Books.
– Paul Wenner, Creator of Gardenburger, author of "Garden Cuisine"

More Americans than ever before say they are suffering from asthma.
It is one of America's most common and costly diseases! – www.aafa.org

Treating Asthma Naturally Brings Results!

Famous Dr. Andrew Weil, stated in his Self Healing Letter, *"I have seen asthma disappear completely in response to major diet shifts such as eliminating sugar, milk products and switching to a healthy vegetarian regime."* Johns Hopkins Medical Studies and others suggest those who monitored their diets to be low in meat, no milk and no additives, were less likely to have asthma problems. Sadly, most doctors believe erroneously there is no cure for asthma. Asthma attacks can be life-threatening. For short-term acute asthma help, bronchodilating drugs (often addictive with side effects) are at times necessary until breathing improves. There are natural remedies that, while not substitutes for bronchodilators, may help manage acute asthma episodes until breathing improves.

Butterbur Root: Studies have shown that patients who treated their asthma with butterbur in addition to prescribed steroids experienced much more freedom of air flow than those who were treated with inhaled steroids alone. Make sure you get the certified PA-free product.

Ginkgo Biloba: has also been used to help patients deal with asthma. This herbal extract helps to block a compound known as PAF, or platelet activating factor, which plays a large role in the flare-ups of asthma symptoms.

83

Lobelia: is used by many naturopathic physicians to treat asthma. Keep on hand a mixture combining three parts tincture of lobelia with one part tincture of capsicum (red pepper). At start of asthmatic attack, take 5-10 drops of mixture in distilled water. As needed repeat every 30-60 minutes up to 4 times for total of 3 or 4 doses.

Eucalyptus Oil: Pure eucalyptus oil is an effective treatment for asthma symptoms because of its decongestant properties. Put 2-3 drops of eucalyptus oil in a pot of boiling water and deeply breathe in the steam.

---

*The beautiful thing about learning is that
no one can take it away from you. – B.B. King*

---

*When you are kind to others, it not only
changes you, it changes the world.
– Harold Kushner, Prominent Rabbi and Author*

For Long Term Control & Prevention of Asthma

- Eliminate sugar and all processed foods. Decrease protein to 20% of daily caloric intake or even better replace animal protein with plant based proteins (avoid soy).

- Eliminate milk and milk products, substituting other calcium sources, such as rice, coconut or almond milk.

- Eat organically grown fruits and vegetables.

- Eliminate polyunsaturated vegetable oils, margarine, vegetable shortening, all partially hydrogenated oils that might contain trans-fatty acids, and all foods that contain trans-fatty acids, such as deep-fried foods.

- Use extra-virgin olive oil as your main fat.

- Increase intake of omega-3's (flaxseeds and walnuts).

- Always drink plenty of distilled water and green juices to keep your respiratory tract secretions more fluid.

- Experiment with eliminating (one at a time) wheat (white flour), corn, soy and sugar for 6-8 weeks to see if the condition improves (keep daily journal – page 146).

- Eat ginger and turmeric for anti-inflammatory effects.

- Have manipulative work done on chest to break up restrictive patterns in nerves and muscles that develop in chronic asthma. Best systems for this are Chest Tapping and Rolfing, a form of deep-tissue massage (page 193).

- Minimize contact with respiratory irritants, such as smoke, dust, molds, and volatile organic compounds (VOC). Remove sources of offending materials from your home or office, install a good air filtration system. Experiment with living in other locations: in high mountains, the desert, or near the seacoast. Asthma may improve greatly with a change of climate.

- In adults, GERD may be an underlying asthma cause. In such cases, successful apple cider vinegar treatment of digestive problems often helps clear up the asthma.

- Experiment with traditional Chinese Medicine and Ayurvedic Medicines. These systems are sometimes able to offer significant help through more specific dietary adjustments and herbal treatments.

- Commit to weekly fasts and detoxification protocols such as lymphatic drainage therapy, colon hydrotherapy and infrared saunas.

- Focus on healing your digestive system by taking food enzymes with meals and practicing food combining.

Info from Dr. Andrew Weil • DrWeil.com

84

What is Bronchitis?

Bronchitis is the inflammation of mucus membranes of the main air passages of the lungs (the bronchial tree comprising the bronchi and the bronchioles). It causes congestion in the chest, coughing, difficulty in breathing and chest tightness. Acute Bronchitis is generally caused by a lung infection, 90% of which are viral in origin. Most Americans with a sore throat or bronchitis are prescribed antibiotics even though just a fraction stand to benefit from them. Almost all sore throats are caused by viruses . . . "so an antibiotic is not going to help and it has a very real chance of hurting you," says Dr. Jeffrey Linder, Research for Brigham and Women's Hospital in Boston*.

Home Remedies to Help Cure Bronchitis

Instead of using antibiotics, here are a few home remedies that come in handy to anyone suffering from bronchitis or any other similar respiratory ailment. Try these remedies during the early stages and see results.

- Eating hot, spicy foods like chili peppers, help thin the mucus in your lungs and help to drain your phlegm.

- Inhaling steam aids in loosening the secretions of the lungs, which drains phlegm. Take a hot shower or breathe in steam from hot boiling water with apple cider vinegar or Oil of Oregano added (page 31). Also try eucalyptus, lavender or peppermint oils (see page 36).

- Avoid alcohol, caffeinated drinks, sugar and processed food, and instead drink plenty of purified water or make apple cider vinegar drink (page 144).

- Mix $1/2$ tsp each of cinnamon, cloves and ground ginger in a cup of boiling water. Stir and cool slightly, then drink it for several days.

- Add $1/2$ tsp of powdered sesame seed in 2 Tbsps of water. Mix it well and take it twice daily.

Antibiotics can have bad side effects, including: stomach pain, severe diarrhea and yeast infections. They can also cause drug-resistant germs – which means future infections could be harder to treat (beware of antibacterial soaps). Antibiotics should only be prescribed if you have strep throat, which is caused by bacteria that could be killed with antibiotics.

– Reuters.com

- Mix crushed almonds in a glass of freshly squeezed orange juice. Regular use of this can help quell respiratory troubles. Vitamin C supplements and fresh fruit juices also help to fight respiratory viruses.
- Boil a few leaves of basil in water and drink it.
- Ginger is a very good remedy for most of the respiratory disorders. Make a tea by adding ½ tsp of freshly grated ginger, ground cloves and ground black pepper and allow to boil. You can sweeten it with honey to help build immunity against diseases and allergies.
- Drink one teaspoon raw onion juice in morning, great remedy for bronchitis and other respiratory infections.

About Chronic Obstructive Pulmonary Disease

In the US the term "COPD" includes two main conditions – *emphysema* and *chronic bronchitis*. Chronic bronchitis is an inflammation of the lining of your bronchial tubes, which carry air to and from your lungs. Emphysema occurs when the air sacs (alveoli) at the end of the smallest air passages (bronchioles) in the lungs are gradually destroyed. Most people who have COPD have both emphysema and chronic bronchitis. Thus, the general term "COPD" is more accurate.

COPD is a major cause of disability and is the 3rd leading cause of death in US. Currently, millions of people are diagnosed with or have COPD unknowingly. The main cause of COPD is tobacco smoking! Other irritants can cause COPD, such as cigar smoke, secondhand smoke, pipe smoke, air pollution and workplace exposure to dust, smoke or fumes. COPD has no cure and doctors don't know how to reverse the damage. However, treatments and lifestyle changes can help you feel better and stay more active and slow the progress of the disease. Info from *www.nhlbi.nih.gov* and *www.mayoclinic.org*

Studies show that using Mullein may help in treating COPD. Laboratory results show that mullein kills viruses on contact in test tubes, and may boost effectiveness of some medications that treat influenza. It can help break up phlegm and soothe irritated mucus membranes. Mullein is available as liquid or dried extract. You can make mullein tea by adding 1-2 tsps. of dried leaves and flowers to 1 cup boiling water and steep for 10 minutes. – LiveStrong.com

COPD Natural Remedies and Treatments

Quit Smoking: According to the American Thoracic Society (ATS), about 90% of people with COPD get the disease from smoking. Quitting is the most important lifestyle change you can make to ease COPD symptoms. Prolonged chronic asthma can progress into lung destructing emphysema.

Stay Active: Staying physically active is the second most important thing you can do at home to help manage symptoms of COPD. According to the Mayo Clinic, regular exercise can actually strengthen your respiratory muscles, improve your breathing and your overall strength and endurance. Try brisk walking, jogging, gardening, golfing, tennis or even shopping (see page 178-179).

Eat Right: Eating healthy foods and maintaining a proper weight can significantly help improve breathing. For more info on eating a healthy diet see pages 121-124.

Control Breathing: Breathing exercises and relaxation techniques can help you breathe more efficiently throughout the day. See Bragg Super Power Breathing Exercises on pages 67-77. These breathing exercises increase your blood oxygen levels and help reduce shortness of breath.

Stay Hydrated: drink plenty of purified water and fruit juices. Use humidifier to keep airways clear of mucus.

Protect Yourself: When you have COPD, it's important to avoid situations that can aggravate your symptoms. Cold air can trigger bronchospasm, a sudden constriction in the muscles of airway walls that leads to shortness of breath! Respiratory infections can cause COPD symptoms to worsen, so wise to stay away from crowds if possible.

Take Care of Your Emotions: The changes in your life caused by COPD and its symptoms may cause you to experience some difficult emotions. Grief, anger, anxiety, and depression are all normal responses to chronic illness.

Reduce Stress: Stress can exacerbate COPD symptoms like shortness of breath, so it's important to manage the level of stress in your life! Take some time each day to unwind, both physically and mentally. You can relax by napping, listening to soothing music, reading quietly, or doing something that you find enjoyable and soothing.

Deep Breathing & The Bragg Healthy Lifestyle Can Revitalize Lungs with More Oxygen

Prolonged chronic asthma can often progress into lung destructing emphysema and COPD. This causes air sacs to become so distended with trapped stale air they lose elasticity, and can slowly suffocate. Bragg Super Power Breathing can't restore destroyed tissue, but it can help salvage and revitalize the rest of the lungs! The life-giving inflow of oxygen acts as a natural decongestant and gradually cleans out bronchioles and bronchial tubes! This helps remove toxic carbon dioxide and other waste from air sacs and lung tissues. This cleansing and opening-up of the lungs helps revitalize every possible cell with more oxygen and nutrients!

Respiratory ailment victims have gained permanent relief by following The Bragg Healthy Lifestyle and eliminating all milk products, ice cream, yogurt, cheese, butter, etc., along with fasting for a 24-hour period weekly and eating a healthy vegetarian live food diet. It's absolutely essential you eliminate all cow's milk and its products from your diet, as these produce mucus and sickness!

Do Bragg Super Power Breathing exercises (pages 67-77), gradually increase walks and exercise. Take vitamin C and E and CoQ10 (see pages 149, 151-153); they promote lung tissue healing and help reduce inflammatory and bronchial wall swelling. Read page 36 for herbs and supplements. Make sure to eat a healthy diet – organic fruits and vegetables, nuts, seeds, whole grains, beans, legumes, etc. (see pages 121-124). Drink 8 glasses of purified/distilled water daily – keeps you hydrated. Make sure you get sufficient sleep – at least 8 hours nightly (see pages 91-94). Get plenty of gentle sunshine and fresh air daily (see pages 187-189). For more info on The Bragg Healthy Lifestyle please read Bragg Books. See back of this book for our other titles.

Next time you go to toss an orange peel, don't! Grate, sprinkle on foods. Organic orange peels are rich powerful flavonoid antioxidants that reduce oxidative damage and fight free radicals! Plus they are loaded with natural histamine – a suppressing compound that can help expel congestion associated with bronchitis, colds and flu. Helps keep lungs cleansed.
– Mike Adams

Important Self-Health Care for Healthy Lungs

Because standard drugs are suppressive in nature, they tend to perpetuate asthma and reduce the chance that it will disappear on its own – especially in children. Try these natural self-care measures to prevent attacks, improve lung health and lessen the need for any drugs.

• **Use a peak-flow meter**, a hand-held device that you can blow into to measure the amount of air in your lungs.

• **Reduce asthma & respiratory triggers** by learning causes and eliminating all destructive triggers from your life.

• **Drink 8-10 glasses of purified/distilled water daily**, to help keep respiratory-tract secretions moist and fluid. Drinking plenty of water speeds process of eliminating irritants and toxins from the body. Avoid dehydration!

• **Supplement your diet daily with 3,000 mg. vitamin C.**

• **Say "no" to milk and dairy products** which increases mucus that worsens asthma and allergies! Web: *NotMilk.com*

• **Change your diet**. Food allergies (pages 37-38) trigger chronic asthma attacks and respiratory-breathing problems.

89

• **Be manipulated.** Go to a Chiropractor or Osteopath and have them check for any restrictions in back, neck, chest and diaphragm areas. A skilled practitioner can free them up. When needed this can help promote healing and health.

• **Exercise wisely.** Warm up slowly with stretching and breathing exercises (at least 10-15 minutes). Don't walk or jog within 50 feet of a heavy traffic road (car fumes are toxic). Enjoy parks with lawns, trees and fresh clean air.

• **Clear the air.** Use HEPA filters (page 115) in rooms or entire house with a filter system and also in your car.

• **Hang some plants** (Spider plants, Boston ferns, English Ivy) in your house, work and office. Plants absorb toxic vapors and gases that help purify the air for your lungs.

• **Relax.** Do breathing exercises and rest (pgs. 67-77, 155-160).

• **Consider healthy healing alternatives** (pages 191-197). Example: a young asthmatic patient was so improved after two months of a Ayurvedic health treatment that he dispensed with most of his medication (pages 44-45).

Mother Nature Loves You To Enjoy Her Beauty

Let me look upward
into the branches
Of the towering oak
And know that it grew
slowly and well.

Give me, amidst
the confusion
of my day
The calmness of the
everlasting hills.

90

Let me pause
to look at a flower,
to smell a rose —
God's autograph,
to chat with a friend,
to read a few lines
from a good book.

Break the tensions
of my nerves
With the soothing music
of singing streams
and gentle rains
That live in
my memory.

Follow steps of the godly,
and stay on the right path
to enjoy life to the fullest.
— Proverbs 2:20-21

Open your eyes to behold wondrous things out of Thy law. – Psalm 119:18

Chapter 14

Sleeping & Snoring Problems

America's National "Sleep Debt"

A National Sleep Foundation poll discovered that a whopping 67% of American adults have a sleeping problem and that over one-third (37%), are so sleepy during the daytime that their daily activities are interfered with. Over the past 100 years, we've reduced our average sleep time by 20% and, over the last 25 years, added an additional month to our annual work/commute time. Our national "sleep debt" is rising and while our society has changed, our physical bodies and needs have not! We are paying dearly for such unhealthy "progress!" Visit their informative website: *www.SleepFoundation.org.*

Are You Getting Enough Sleep Lately?

The odds are you are not getting sufficient sleep. American adults presently average 7 hours nightly. While everyone's sleep needs vary, most scientific research indicates that we require 8 hours of sleep nightly. Few are lucky enough to enjoy 5 to 6 hours of sound sleep and still perform well at work. To just get "caught up," a full ten hours of rest, plus naps are frequently called for!!!

First make a clear choice about how you wish to spend the 30-45 minutes that precede your actual going to bed. Avoid a rush to "get things ready for tomorrow" or to catch up on tasks not completed during the day. This is a time to relax and rest your body and mind. Try an aroma herbal bath or a self-massage (with olive oil) while showering, one hour before bed – it's so relaxing. Enjoy a warm soothing apple cider vinegar drink with cinnamon and honey (recipe on page 144) or a Lemon Balm or Sleepytime herbal tea before bedtime. Lemon Balm, whose scientific name is *melissa officinalis,* is a soothing plant with both nervine and antiseptic, relaxing natural qualities. It's a member of the peppermint and spearmint family and is grown worldwide. When flowering it has a lemon fragrance – a perfume delight.

Good Sleep is a Cornerstone of Good Health

Eight hours nightly is the optimal amount of sleep for most adults! Science has established that a sleep deficit can have serious, far reaching effects on your health!

Interrupted or Lack of Proper Sleep Can:

- Dramatically weaken your immune system
- Accelerate tumor growth with severe sleep dysfunctions
- Cause a pre-diabetic state, making you feel hungry and then you over-fuel your body causing obesity
- Seriously impair your memory. Even a single night of poor sleep (4-6 hours) can impact your ability to think clearly
- Impair your performance on physical or mental tasks
- Also increase stress-related disorders including: heart disease, stomach ulcers, constipation, mood disorders, personality upsets and depression

Healthful Tips for Sound, Recharging Sleep
Excerpts from Dr. Mercola – www.mercola.com

92 "The good news is there are many natural techniques you can learn to restore your "sleep health." Whether you have difficulty falling asleep or feel inadequately rested when waking up, you can find some relief from the tips below:

• **Sleep in complete darkness.** Even the tiniest bit of light in the room can disrupt your internal clock and your pineal gland's production of melatonin and serotonin. Little bits of light pass directly through your optic nerve to your hypothalamus, which controls your biological clock. Light signals your brain that it's time to wake up and starts preparing your body for ACTION!!!

• **Wear an eye mask to block out light.** It is not always easy to block out every stream of light using curtains or blinds.

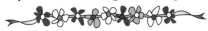

The average person spends about 24 years of a 78 year lifespan asleep.

A recharging, peaceful good night sleep is vitally important!

 "No external conditions are required for happiness. Happiness is who you are!"
—Dr. Jay Kumar

• **Keep your bedroom at a lower temp (60-65°F is best) for sleeping.** Scientists believe a cooler bedroom is most conducive to sleep since it mimics body's natural temperature drop.

• **Check bedroom for Electro-Magnetic Fields (EMFs).** EMF's can disrupt pineal gland and production of melatonin and serotonin. To check this you will need a gauss meter. Before going to bed unplug any phones, clocks or radios near bed. Even when in hotels. (see below)

• **Move alarm clocks and other electric devices away from your bed.** It adds to your worry when you stare at it all night – 2 am – 3 am – 4:30 am. Prior to use of electricity, people would go to bed shortly after sundown and then rise with the sun as most animals do. Mother Nature intended this for humans as well.

• **Get to bed as early as possible.** Your body recharges between the hours of 11 pm and 1 am. Also, your gallbladder dumps toxins during this same period. If you are awake, the toxins back up into your liver, which can further disrupt your sleep and your health.

• **Establish bedtime routine.** Try meditation, prayer, deep breathing, aromatherapy, essential oils or a massage.

• **It is best not to drink fluids 2 hours before bedtime.** This helps reduce frequency of needing to go to bathroom. Also make sure you **empty your bladder right before bed.**

• **Have a high-protein drink/shake several hours before bed.** This helps provide L-tryptophan needed for your melatonin and serotonin production (SlimFast, Ensure).

Is Electro-Magnetic (EM) Energy Hurting You?

A wide array of symptoms have been attributed to EM exposure. Many complain of: headaches, dizziness, memory loss, irritability, depression, anxiety, fatigue, muscle and joint pain, spasms, numbness, paralysis, strokes, insomnia, heart palpitations, irregular heartbeat, increased blood pressure, shortness of breath, sinus problems, asthma, bronchitis, shortness of breath, pain or burning of the eyes, blurred vision, cataracts, skin rash, flushing itching, teeth pain, nosebleeds, hair loss, ringing in the ears, thyroid illness. It has been suggested, but not confirmed, that cell phones kept in your pants are linked to testicular cancer and lower sperm counts. Try not to live or work close to high-tension electric wires, TV stations, or cell phone towers. The best thing to do if you are seriously ill is to check out other areas that do not cause symptoms. If some areas of your town are badly polluted with high-tension wires or other sources of EM Energy it is best to cut your losses and move to a place where you feel fine as soon as possible.
Nothing is as important as retaining or regaining your health.

- **Avoid before bed snacks** (particularly grains & sugars).

- **Take a hot bath, shower or sauna before bed.** The temperature drop from getting out of the bath or shower helps to signal your body it's time for bed and sleep.

- **Wear socks to bed.** Study shows wearing socks reduces night wakings. You could put hot water in glass bottle at feet at night. It's so comforting.

- **Put work away at least one hour before bed.** This gives your mind a chance to unwind so you can go to sleep feeling calm, not hyped up or anxious about tomorrow's deadlines.

- **No TV one hour before bed.** TV disrupts your pineal gland function.

- **Keep a Daily Journal.** (page 146) Write in morning when brain is functioning at its peak and cortisol levels are high."

Lifestyle Suggestions That Enhance Sleep

- Avoid stimulants: caffeine (in coffee, some teas, even green teas, soft drinks, chocolate, sugar) and nicotine (found in cigarettes and other tobacco products).

- Don't drink alcohol to "help" you sleep, it's unhealthy!

- Have herbal teas – anise, lemon balm, Sleepytime, chamomile (beware some Green Teas have caffeine), or try melatonin, tryptophan (5HTP), valerian, calcium and magnesium supplements; they work miracles.

- Exercise regularly, but try to be finished with your workout no sooner than 2 hours prior to bedtime.

- Avoid foods you may be sensitive to. Reactions can cause excess congestion, gastrointestinal upset, bloating or gas.

- Associate your bed with recharging sleep – it's best not to sit on it to work or watch TV. *Try a memory 2" foam topper (so comfortable) on your firm mattress.*

- If you suffer from insomnia, don't nap during the day. Remember, earn better sleep by exercise and day activity.

Humor and Laughter are healthy – they improve blood circulation, boost immune system, and help relieve stress.
– Dr. Joel Goodman, author "Laffirmations"

Nervous Tension can ruin your health in dozens of ways and diminish your productivity and even shorten lifespan. – Dr. E. Jacobson, "You Must Relax"

Get Peaceful Sleep – Stop Snoring

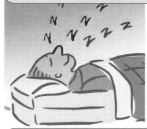

If snoring is happening frequently it can affect the quantity and quality of your sleep and that of family members. Snoring can lead to poor sleep, daytime fatigue, irritability, and increased health problems.

Where Does Snoring Come From?

People who snore often have too much throat and nasal tissue, or "floppy" tissue that is more prone to vibrate. The position of your tongue can also get in the way of smooth breathing. Snoring happens when you can't move air freely through your nose and mouth during sleep, often caused by narrowing of your airway, either from poor sleep posture or abnormalities of the soft tissues in your throat. A narrow airway impairs smooth breathing and creates the sound of snoring.

Common Causes of Snoring

Not all snoring is the same. Everyone snores for different reasons. When you understand why you snore, then you can better find the right solutions to a quieter sleep.

Age. As you reach middle age, your throat becomes narrower, and the muscle tone in your throat decreases.

The way you're built. Men have narrower air passages than women and are more likely to snore! A narrow throat, cleft palate, enlarged adenoids, obesity and other physical attributes which may be hereditary can contribute to snoring.

Nasal and sinus problems. Blocked airway passages with mucus, can make breathing difficult and can create a vacuum in the throat, which can lead to snoring.

Being overweight or out of shape. Obesity, fatty tissue and poor body muscle tone can contribute to snoring.

Alcohol, smoking, and medications. Drinking alcohol, smoking, and certain medications can increase throat muscle relaxation which can lead to more snoring.

Sleep posture. Sleeping flat on back can cause flesh of throat to relax and block airway. Use head cradle pillow.

Is It Snoring or Is It Sleep Apnea?

Snoring could indicate sleep apnea, a potentially life-threatening condition that requires medical attention. Sleep apnea is a breathing obstruction, causing the sleeper to keep waking up to begin breathing again. Normal snoring doesn't interfere with the quality of your sleep as much as sleep apnea, so if you're suffering from extreme fatigue and sleepiness during the day, your problem may be more than just snoring. Please seek medical advice (for more info on sleep apnea please read pages 98-100).

How You Snore Reveals Why You Snore

It's crucial to note different ways you sleep and snore! Sleep positions reveal a lot, and figuring out how you snore can reveal why you snore! Observing patterns in your snoring can often help pinpoint reasons why you snore, what makes it worse, and how to go about stopping your snoring.

• *Closed-mouth snoring* may indicate problem with tongue.

• *Open-mouth snoring* may be related to tissues in throat.

• *Snoring when sleeping on your back* is probably mild snoring. Start improving sleep habits and living The Bragg Healthy Lifestyle for the best and most effective cures.

• *Snoring in all sleep positions* can mean snoring is more severe and may require a more comprehensive treatment.

Some Self-Help Cures To Stop Snoring

There are many things you can do on your own to help you stop snoring. Home remedies and lifestyle changes can go a long way in resolving snoring health problems.

Lose weight. Losing even a little bit of weight can reduce the fatty tissue in the back of the throat and can help decrease or even stop your snoring.

Exercise can also help. Working out to tone your arms, legs, and abs, for example, also leads to toning the muscles in your throat, which in turn can lead to less snoring.

Quit smoking. If you smoke, chances of snoring and cancer are high. Smoking causes airways to be blocked by irritating membranes in the throat, sinus and nose.

Avoid alcohol, sleeping pills, and sedatives, especially before bedtime, because they relax the muscles in the throat and interfere with breathing. Talk to your doctor about any medications you're taking, as some encourage a deeper level of sleep which can make snoring worse.

Bedtime Remedies To Help You Stop Snoring

Clear nasal passages. Having a stuffy nose makes inhalation difficult and creates a vacuum in your throat, which can lead to snoring. Try nasal strips to help you breathe more easily while sleeping (pages 35-36).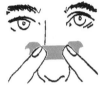

Keep bedroom air moist with a humidifier. Dry air can irritate membranes in the nose and throat.

Reposition your neck. Elevating your head four inches may ease breathing and encourage your tongue and jaw to move forward. There are specially designed cradle pillows to help prevent snoring by making sure your neck and throat muscles are not crimped.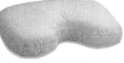

Memory Foam Pillows

Avoid caffeine, heavy meals and drinking within 2 hours of going to bed, especially dairy products.

Sleep on your side. Avoid sleeping flat on your back, as gravity makes it more likely for your tongue and soft tissues to drop and obstruct your airway.

A Different Kind of Relief for Snorer in the House

There are choices in treatments for relieving stubborn snoring. A simple doctor laser treatment could be the answer, or try – RIPSNORE™. A simple, one-piece device that molds to the shape of your mouth. The device is very flexible when being fitted. It stops snoring or drastically reduces snoring in 98% of people who use it. The RIPSNORE™ holds your lower jaw slightly forward, moving the base of the tongue away from the back of airway and soft palate – allowing the throat to be opened and snores to be silenced. The device is almost identical to dental ones. *www.ripsnore.com.au*

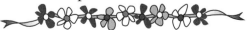

Happiness is a rainbow in your heart – a real health sparkler!
– Patricia Bragg

Somnoplasty: An Effective Treatment For Blocked Nasal Airways, Snoring & Sleep Apnea

Somnoplasty is a minimally invasive procedure that can be performed as an in-office surgery. It is done under local anesthesia with typical time lasting 15-20 minutes. The procedure involves using radio frequency heat to shrink relevant tissues leading to the shrinkage of inner tissues. For chronic nasal obstruction – the turbinates are targeted; habitual snoring the soft palate and uvula; and sleep apnea the base of the tongue and other airway structures.

What Is Sleep Apnea?

Sleep apnea is a sleep disorder in which you have pauses in breathing or shallow breaths while you sleep. Breathing pauses can last from a few seconds to minutes. They often occur 5-30 times or more an hour. Typically, normal breathing then starts again. When you stop breathing, the balance of oxygen and carbon dioxide in the blood is upset. This imbalance stimulates the brain to restart the breathing process. The brain signals you to wake up so that the muscles of the tongue and throat can increase the size of the airway. Then, carbon dioxide can escape and oxygen can enter the airway. These waking episodes are necessary to restart breathing (and to save your life). You may not remember them, but they do disrupt sleep and can cause daytime exhaustion.

Effects of Sleep Apnea on Your Health

Sleep apnea has serious health consequences and can be life-threatening. Please seek medical advice if you think you have sleep apnea. The main effects of sleep apnea are sleep and oxygen deprivation. With your breathing spurts your brain does not get enough oxygen. Problems can result from not getting enough oxygen, including: slow reflexes, poor concentration, and an increased risk of accidents. Also, heart disease, high blood pressure, stroke, diabetes, sexual dysfunction, weight gain and learning and memory problems (see box on page 92).

Sleep Apnea Signs and Symptoms

It can be tough to identify sleep apnea on your own, since most prominent symptoms only occur when you're asleep (you can try recording yourself during sleep). But some of the major signs and symptoms of sleep apnea are:

Pauses that occur while you snore, and if choking or gasping follows the pauses, these are major signs that you have sleep apnea! These breathing pauses typically last between 10-20 seconds and can occur up to hundreds of times a night, jolting you out of your natural sleep rhythm.

Another common sleep apnea sign is fighting sleepiness during the day, at work, or while driving. You may find yourself rapidly falling asleep during the quiet moments of the day when you're not active. Other common signs and symptoms of sleep apnea are:

- *Morning headaches*
- *Memory, learning and concentration problems*
- *Feeling irritable, depressed, or having mood swings*
- *Waking up frequently at night to urinate*
- *Dry mouth or sore throat when you wake up*

99

Some of the Risk Factors For Sleep Apnea

You have a higher risk for sleep apnea if you are:

- Overweight
- Male
- A smoker
- Related to someone who has sleep apnea
- Over the age of 65

Other risk factors include certain physical attributes, such as having a thick neck, deviated septum, receding chin, or enlarged tonsils or adenoids (the most common cause of sleep apnea in children). Your airway may be blocked or narrowed during sleep simply because your throat muscles tend to relax more than normal. Allergies or other medical conditions that cause nasal congestion and blockage can also contribute to sleep apnea.

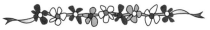

Help me to know the magic of rest and relaxation and restoring power of sleep.
– From poem "Slow Me Down, Lord" – Hittite prayer dating back 2000 years

Self-Help Treatment for Sleep Apnea

While a diagnosis of sleep apnea can be scary, it is a treatable condition! Minor sleep apnea is responsive to most self-health remedies, especially a healthy lifestyle. Some of the following treatments for sleep apnea might work for you:

1. **Lose Weight:** by losing even 10%, you can often help reduce sleep apnea and improve your sleep quality.

2. **Stop using alcohol, tobacco and sedatives:** these relax the muscles of the throat, also encouraging snoring.

3. **Sleep on your side:** those who have apnea usually experience sleep apnea when they sleep flat on back.

4. **Elevate the head of your bed 4 to 6 inches:** This can help alleviate snoring and make breathing easier.

5. **Maintain regular sleep hours.** Sticking to a steady sleep schedule will help you relax and sleep better. Apnea episodes decrease when you get plenty of sleep.

6. **Use a nasal dilator,** *BreatheRight*® **Nasal Strips or make a saline wash squeeze bottle** to help keep nasal passages open.

100

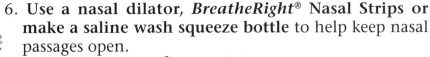

Healthy Mind Habit:

Wake up and say – Today I am going to be happier, healthier and wiser in my daily living! I am the captain of my life and am going to steer it to living a 100% healthy lifestyle! Fact is happy people look younger and have fewer health problems! – Patricia Bragg, Pioneer Health Crusader

Everyone has a doctor within himself. We just have to help it in its work. The natural healing force within each one of us is the greatest force in getting well! – Hippocrates, Father of Medicine, 400 B.C.

Slow, deep breathing and relaxation techniques are important health benefits to the entire body's system. Such techniques as sitting quietly, ignoring distracting thoughts, meditating and praying can bring down blood pressure and these healthy habits have no side effects. – Harvard Health Letter

Lavender helps you relax! Before drying off after evening or nightly bath or shower, place three drops of lavender essential oil on a damp washcloth and rub it gently over your body. The soothing active agents in lavender oil will enter body through your skin and nose.

Chapter 15

Unhealthy Buildings and Homes Cause Many Breathing and Health Problems

Unhealthy

Healthy

Because we human beings have managed to pollute the water, air, and earth, our Mother Nature suffers! We know now that to stay healthy we must take precautions in some areas when we go in to the great outdoors – or even in our backyard! But, it is probably a surprise to most people that even the "great indoors" can be unhealthy and polluted also! Studies show many homes and buildings are so toxic they are unfit to live in and work in.

Today, unfortunately, many modern homes, buildings, and even new cars (page 103) that protect us from the elements, contain invisible toxic vapors that cause health problems as they give shelter! Contamination sources are many – and sadly often far too unrecognized and unaddressed!

101

Beware of Toxic Building Materials

Toxic building materials are the major source of environmental contaminants inside our homes, schools and places of business! For years unknowing builders have used many dangerous substances! Building materials, such as particle board, asbestos, and treated wood, can pose serious health threats. Other deadly substances include **roofing materials** and **insulation** – especially those made with **formaldehyde**, because they leak poisonous vapors! In addition, the horrors of **lead paint** (*www.epa.gov/lead*) still threaten many people living in older homes. Lead is a highly toxic metal that may cause a range of health problems, especially in young children! When lead is absorbed into the body, it can cause damage to the brain and other vital organs, like the kidneys, nerves and blood.

Pollutants may negatively react chemically with body's tissues. – Dr. Andrew Weil

Formaldehyde Gives Off Toxic Vapors

Above your head, under your feet, on and in your walls, all around you in your home, formaldehyde could be poisoning your home and you. Formaldehyde is a colorless, strong-smelling gas. It is used to make building materials and household products. Formaldehyde is used to make walls, cabinets and furniture. Many contractors continue to use this toxic chemical as a preservative, binding agent and insulator. It turns up everywhere in our homes and buildings. Despite its widespread use, we know that formaldehyde is an eye, nose, throat and skin irritant – and is a strong suspected carcinogen! Formaldehyde can make you sick if you breathe it in too much. Symptoms can include: sore throat, cough, scratchy eyes and nosebleeds. Other symptoms include upper respiratory illnesses and allergies. **Formaldehyde is known to cause cancer.** Formaldehyde can irritate the airways, so people with asthma, bronchitis, or other breathing conditions are especially sensitive to toxic formaldehyde. See web: *Cancer.gov/CancerTopics/FactSheet/Risk/Formaldehyde*

102 How do you cure your house of formaldehyde sickness? Unfortunately little can be done unless you build your house from scratch with careful attention to using only safe, natural building materials! Beyond this, only time will purify and heal the sick home. Over many years the toxic residues in building materials emit less harmful vapors, making older homes healthier homes – and the people who live there can become healthier too.

Beware of Invisible Radon Gas Dangers

Like formaldehyde, radon is an invisible killer lurking in many homes, buildings and soil. Radon is a cancer-causing radioactive gas. You cannot see, smell or taste radon, but it may be a problem in your home. The Surgeon General has warned that radon is the second leading cause of lung cancer in the United States today. If you smoke and your home has high radon levels, you're at a high risk for developing lung cancer!

Be your own Health Captain and do what needs to be done for your health!

Although not much can be done, it's important to find out if your home has radon contamination! Contact your local health department and ask if you live in high radon area. If you have concerns, ask to have a radon test done in your home and surrounding area. Also natural stones and bricks used in construction should be checked for radon. Ask about remedial actions. If your home has high radon levels, seriously consider moving to a healthy home.

Check this website for radon info:
www.radon.com

Beware of Toxic Dangerous VOCs "Off-Gassing"

Off-gassing is the evaporation of toxic chemicals from: furniture, plastics, vinyl products, paints, office printers, cleaners and soaps, new car vapors, new clothing, cosmetics, mattresses, carpets, plywood and more. **Off-gassing emits Volatile Organic Compounds (VOCs)**, silent poisonous gasses and small particulate substances often throughout the life of the material.

What about **synthetic carpets**? That soft carpeting that feels cozy under your feet is constantly shedding toxic vapors into your home. Carpets can emit VOCs for five years or possibly more, although the off-gassing decreases significantly several months after installation. The Environmental Protection Agency advises ventilating well for at least 72 hours after installation by opening windows and using fans that move air directly to the outdoors. Crawling toddlers are the most vulnerable!

103

The U.S. Environmental Protection Agency (EPA) and Surgeon General's Office have estimated that as many as 20,000 lung cancer deaths are caused each year by radon. Radon-induced lung cancer costs United States over $2 billion dollars per year in both direct and indirect health care costs. – radon.com

A merry heart is good medicine; but a broken spirit destroys health. "A merry heart is healthful, but one that is broken in spirit and dejected will develop many bodily illnesses. Nothing ruins health faster than grief, anger, bad temper, jealousy, hatred, anxiety, worry and malice. We should cleanse and rid ourselves of all bad habits." – Proverbs 17:22

Health and cheerfulness naturally beget each other. – Joseph Addison

Healthy Home Environment is Important Check for Lead, Radon and Formaldehyde

Who wants to be sick and live in a sick home? You make the effort to eat well, sleep well and get exercise, don't drop the ball when it comes to ensuring a healthy living environment! **Here are some playing-it-safe ideas:**

First, be sure you and your family are safe from the dangers of *radon.* **Second,** be safe from the dangers of *formaldehyde*; older homes usually have less. However, radon contamination is often worse in older homes. **Third,** be safe from the dangers of *lead paint* which is greater in older homes. Test for all three when considering a home. **Have a licensed home inspector check for all three toxins** and others that might be sickening your home or building you will plan to live in. **It's reasonable and important!**

Don't cover floors with *toxic carpeting.* If you must put something on wood floors, the safest choices are carpets and area rugs made from natural materials, wool or cotton. Don't cook with gas in an *unventilated room.* Be sure that your gas flame burns a clean blue. If you cook in a closed room with an orange flame you and your house will suffer from carbon dioxide, carbon monoxide, and other toxins.

To make a safe, happy and healthy home, spend the money to equip your house with plenty of windows and doors! Remember what the good doctor said for centuries: *Plenty of clean, fresh air is one of the best cures!* Keep your house well ventilated so that there can never be a poisonous buildup of dangerous toxins! Poisons are often carried around the home by dust particles so **it's wise to buy a home air purifier that removes these toxic particles too.**

MORE ON LEAD PAINT: Lead is a toxic metal that can cause serious health problems if ingested or if dust containing lead is inhaled. Lead has been used in a wide variety of products found in and around our homes, including paint, ceramics, pipes and plumbing materials, gasoline, batteries, ammunition, and cosmetics. Up until 1978, when federal regulations restricted the use of lead in household paint, lead was a common component in exterior and interior paints. Lead can affect almost every organ and system in your body. Even low levels of lead in the blood of children can result in: behavior and learning problems; lower IQ and hyperactivity; slowed growth; hearing problems; and anemia.

Toxic Chemicals Found In Your Home

Many toxic chemicals from household products can be found right in your home. Products such as detergent, floor and furniture polish, paints, various cleaning products for glass, wood, metal, ovens, toilets and drains often contain toxic chemicals and vapors. Air fresheners can contain chemicals harmful to your health. These chemicals may include: ammonia, sulfuric and phosphoric acids, lye, chlorine, formaldehyde, petroleum solvents, and chlorinated phenols! If you have children also consider their art supplies, such as markers, paint and glue. Home furnishings, such as carpets, curtains, wall decorations, and some furniture may be treated with chemicals that are potentially dangerous.

Cleaning Supplies Can Affect Your Health

Many cleaning supplies and household products can irritate your eyes, throat, cause headaches and other health problems. Some products release dangerous chemicals or gasses (vapors), including volatile organic compounds (VOCs). Other harmful ingredients include ammonia and bleach. *CAUTION: Never mix bleach with ammonia – the gasses created from this combination can lead to death! Please read all labels – it could save your life!* Even natural fragrances such as citrus (bathroom sprays often have citrus) can produce dangerous vapor pollutants in your home.

VOCs and other chemicals released when using cleaning supplies contribute to chronic respiratory problems, allergic reactions and headaches. Studies confirm these chemicals affect people who have asthma and other respiratory illnesses.

Products containing toxic VOCs and other toxic substances can include: aerosol spray products, including health, beauty and cleaning products; air fresheners; chlorine bleach; detergent and dish-washing liquids; dry cleaning chemicals; rug and upholstery cleaners; furniture and floor polish; and oven cleaners.

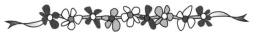

Love begins by taking care of the loved ones at home. – Mother Teresa

Chemicals, Toxic Vapors and Your Health

Each of us react differently to the chemical stew we face on a daily basis, and recognizing such health effects may be difficult! Typical reactions to new carpet VOCs include headaches, nausea, dizziness, shortness of breath, and asthmatic reactions. Longer-term effects are also possible. The CHE (Collaborative on Health and the Environment – see below) lists benzene as having a strong link to leukemia and lymphomas, while styrene is associated with cognitive impairment and hearing loss, among other conditions. (web: *EcologyCenter.org*)

Here are some rules for minimizing VOCs in your home: Buy used goods if possible, the VOCs associated with their production have diminished over time, especially with cars, mattresses and furniture. Choose options like low-or no-VOC paint, which is now widely available and fairly economical! Always stay away from polyvinyl chloride, which is commonly found in linoleum, upholstery, and shower curtains.

An amazing resource – The ***Collaborative on Health and the Environment (CHE) Toxicant and Disease Database*** (*HealthAndEnvironment.org*) is a searchable online database that summarizes links between chemical contaminants and approximately 180 human diseases or conditions. The CHE points out that more than 80,000 chemicals have been developed, distributed, and discarded into the environment over the past 60 years. Most have not been tested for toxic effects in humans or animals, and many are common in our air, water, food, homes, work places, and the communities we live in.

STEPS TO REDUCE EXPOSURE OF VOC's: Increase ventilation when using products that emit VOCs. Make sure to use household products according to manufacturer's directions. Discard unused or little-used containers safely. Buy in quantities that you will use soon. Keep out of reach of children and pets. Never mix household care products unless directed on label. – www.epa.gov

---

Chemicals play a major role in our lives. They are part of what we eat, where we work and how we live. Despite their prevalence in our lives, many chemicals are toxic. Toxic chemicals can be found in our soil, water, air, and bodies. Contaminations seriously effect the health of humans, pets and wildlife everywhere. – www.CEHN.org

Buy Healthy & Safe Products For Your Home

By cleaning out the toxins in your home, just like cleaning out toxins in our bodies, we create a space where energy can flow more easily. Replace toxic products with new improved eco-friendly ones that really work! Some of the worst and most common toxic offenders to watch out for are:

Ammonia – in window and other cleaners. Ammonia can cause coughing, wheezing, nasal complaints, eye irritation, throat discomfort and skin problems. A study showed mice suffered from swelling and bleeding in lungs after 6 weeks of exposure. **Alternatives:** We use white vinegar.

Chlorine – in water, bleach and cleaners – attacks organic matter (you are organic), skin and is a mucous membrane irritant. **Alternatives:** In shower use chlorine-removing shower filter, and use hydrogen peroxide-based bleaches.

Formaldehyde – in new furniture and carpeting – human carcinogen, causes birth defects, asthma and headaches. **Alternatives:** Seek old beautiful furniture available at moving sales and thrift stores. Buy old oriental rugs on *eBay*. They last so much longer and save you money in the long run.

Anti-bacterial soaps – used in bathrooms and at work – breed stronger, more dangerous bacteria by only killing weaker bacteria. **Alternative:** Use Castile all-natural soaps.

Asthma Linked to Home Environment

Over 25 million Americans experience frightening attacks of wheezing and breathlessness that are sometimes fatal. Asthma is not just one disease. Sometimes it's from an allergy and sometimes it's food related. Studies show Asthma is tied to what's inside your home, toxic products, sprays, etc., as well as in your genes, from childhood infections, diet, milk, sugars, fast foods, and even stress! See pages 81-84 for more information on asthma and how to treat it naturally for miracle healings!

Two healthy substitutes to use for household cleansers, deodorizers and disinfectants are baking soda and white vinegar. For safe, non-toxic formulas, techniques and products for cleaning check this web: learn.eartheasy.com

Enjoy Having a Healthy, Safe Home and More

Ensuring that your home is a healthy and safe space for you and your family is not an easy task. But what job could be more rewarding than health, happiness, vitality and a long, productive life? Creating a healthy home might not be inexpensive. However the savings in health care costs, lost productivity, worry and stress will greatly outweigh the short-term costs of making your home a safe haven. **Your home should be your Shangri-la health retreat.**

After you've done what you can about toxic walls and vapors, carpets and appliances here are more suggestions to help reduce your home's toxicity. Read labels of all cleaning products, sprays, etc. Most are full of toxic ingredients, this includes detergents, soaps, fabric softeners, polishes, upholstery, carpet, oven cleaners and air fresheners. Using toxic household cleansers, bug sprays and moth balls, etc. can expose people to harmful vapors! Beware of ammonia, turpentine, paint, acetone, chlorine, sodium hydroxide, bleach, gasoline and all toxic vapors. If you need to use any of these substances, consider only safe, non-toxic, natural versions!

Important To Use Safe Pest and Weed Control

Pesticides and weed control products used around the home can cause a vast array of health problems! If pesticide sprays are being applied in your area, do the following:

1. Go to another section of town for 24-48 hours.
2. Do not allow pets or children outside on the lawn for at least 24 hours after the spraying.
3. If you must stay home, close all doors and windows and turn off air conditioning. If sensitive, seal these.
4. Use a fan in bedroom (mosquitoes do not like a breeze).

Researchers are looking at many irritants – like latex, which sloughs off automobile tires as tiny particles that may end up in your lungs. Some city studies pinpointed cockroaches as key allergens. Energy conservation has locked us in sick, "tight" closed-up office buildings and homes with sick, stale air, environmental toxins, gas appliances, secondhand smoke, pet hair and dander, mites, mold, and bacteria-laden dust.

Chapter 16

Air Pollution & Smog

The urgent problems of air pollution.

These days it doesn't matter where in the world you live or where you go, you can no longer absolutely escape exposure to the poisons that we humans have mindlessly dumped into our air, water and land. In pristine Minnesota, your water might be dangerously contaminated from upstream paper pulp mills. On beautiful New Guinea beaches, you might have to step around hazardous garbage carried great distances by ocean tides. Toxic waste by-products from oil production are found everywhere in the Middle East Deserts.

What these places all have in common from India to Mexico, from California to London and China, is air pollution! This is the greatest toxic scourge of modern man. Some areas are far worse than others. Smoke contamination of the early industrial revolution compared to today's more deadly toxic chemical revolution is almost out of control! When air pollution toxins can actually be seen, it is called *smog*.

109

What Is Smog?

Smog is a general term that refers to the various kinds of visible air pollution! The word *smog* – a combination of the words *smoke* and *fog* – was first invented in Glasgow, Scotland in the early 1900's. It described the thick, bad air that plagued and continues to plague the city. This smog killed over 1,000 people in 1909! Smog today is more complex than simply smoke mixed with fog. Many of these toxic deadly pollutants are invisible to the eye. Reread pages 101-106. Visit *www.epa.gov* or *www.arb.ca.gov*

According to the EPA, cars and trucks contribute more than 50% of the locally-generated air pollution. The remainder comes from solvent evaporation, surface cleaning and coating, petroleum production and other mobile sources (boats, trains, planes), combustion engines and other miscellaneous sources.

Pure, clean air is the invisible staff of life! Smog is an invisible staff of death!

Ground-level Ozone is Deadly Health Hazard

Breathing smoggy air can be hazardous because smog contains ozone, a pollutant that can harm our health when there are elevated levels in the air we breathe. Ozone is a colorless gas composed of three atoms of oxygen. Ozone can be good or bad, depending on where it is found:

Good Ozone: occurs naturally in the Earth's upper atmosphere – 1 to 30 miles above the Earth's surface – where it forms a protective layer that guards plant and animal life from the sun's damaging ultraviolet radiation.

Bad Ozone: in the Earth's lower atmosphere, near ground level, ozone is formed when industrial pollutants emitted by cars, power plants, industrial boilers, refineries, chemical plants and other sources react with sunlight and a dangerous chemical reaction occurs! At ground-level, where we eat, breathe and live, ozone combined with pollutants is responsible for smog's trademark "haze." This has a smothering toxic effect on the city dweller on smoggy days causing choking, coughing and eye-burning. Bad, high ozone concentrations are especially harmful to children, the elderly, those with respiratory illnesses and people who exercise outdoors in smog.

Ground-level Ozone: a key component of smog, damages human lungs and body, animals, crops, even buildings and paint. Scientists have been studying the effects of ozone on human health for many years! (*epa.gov/GroundLevelOzone*) Studies show Ozone promotes dangerous health effects:

1. *Ozone can irritate the entire respiratory system.* You might start coughing and feel irritation in your throat, and experience an uncomfortable sensation in your chest.

2. *Ozone can reduce lung function.* It is more difficult for you to breathe as deeply and vigorously as you normally would.

3. *Ozone can aggravate asthma.* Ozone makes people more sensitive to allergens and reduces your lung function.

4. *Ozone can inflame and damage the lining of the lungs.*

5. *Ozone has many other effects on people's health,* such as chronic lung disease, emphysema and bronchitis. Ozone may reduce the immune system's ability to fight off bacterial infections in the entire respiratory system.

Dirty Air Costs Our Country Billions Annually

Clean air is a delicate balance of Nitrogen (78%), Oxygen (20%), with small amounts of Argon (1%), Carbon Dioxide (.03%), and traces of Neon, Helium, Methane, Krypton, and Sulfur Dioxide. Gases such as carbon dioxide, methane and sulfur dioxide are normal components of clean air – it is when they reach much higher and dangerous concentrations that makes the air polluted and harmful to the environment and human life!

Air pollution is one of the world's biggest health risks, linked to 7 million deaths across the globe yearly, according to the World Health Organization (WHO). Outdoor pollution (from traffic fumes and coal-burning) and indoor pollution (from wood and coal stoves), kills more people than smoking, road deaths and diabetes combined. In the U.S., air pollution causes about 200,000 early deaths a year, with emissions from vehicle transport and power generation as the biggest culprits. California suffers the most air pollution compared to other states. Exposure to "dirty" air can cause premature death, hospitalizations and respiratory symptoms, chronic and acute bronchitis and asthma. It can be limiting to a person's normal daily activity and increases childrens' school absences and lost workdays.

"Dirty" air is not only harmful for human life, it's harmful to the U.S. environment. The harm done to U.S. crops by sulphur dioxide alone is estimated at more than $500 million yearly plus damage done by countless poisons we pour into rivers and seas in terms of reduced fish catches is colossal! Mercury alone is considered responsible for an annual $1 billion's-worth of damage worldwide.

Premature ageing is a highly toxic condition caused by shallow breathing, toxic air, nutritional deficiencies, negative thinking and an unhealthy lifestyle!

California fights carcinogens in the air. Among the chemicals cited are benzene, carbon tetrachloride, chloroform and vinyl chloride. Carcinogens are released into the atmosphere from industries, and autos, especially diesel trucks. Regulations are aimed at these sources.

Breathing pure, clean air deeply gives you more energy, go-power and sparkles up your life. – Patricia Bragg, Health Crusader

Smog Affects Humans, Plants, Animals, Buildings

Pollution not only affects humans by destroying their respiratory, cardiovascular and neurological systems; it also affects nature, plants, fruits, vegetables, rivers, ponds, forests, bees and animals – all of which we highly depend on for survival. Smog impacts the environment by killing innumerable animal species and green life as they strive to adapt to breathing and surviving in such toxic environments. It's crucial to control pollution as nature, wildlife and bees are precious gifts to all mankind. See web: *www.conserve-energy-future.com*

When components of smog – sulphur dioxide, nitrogen oxides and ammonia, end up in plants, surface water and soils, this has a number of toxic consequences:

- Availability of nutrients through soil is likely to decrease.

- When acidity is high then more metals will dissolve in water. This can cause surface water to become polluted, which has serious health effects on aquatic plants, fish and animals. Example: Mercury can be dispersed by transport through surface water, causing it to accumulate in fish.

- Smog can damage all plant life by inhibiting plants' natural ability to make and store food through photosynthesis. When this process is compromised, plant growth, reproduction and the general health of the plant suffers! Smog can weaken plants that are already sensitive and make them more susceptible to infections, diseases, habitat stressers and pests! As a consequence, plants can dry out and become unable to contribute to the greater ecosystem that they belong to. Smog can deplete agricultural crops such as vegetables, soybeans, wheat, tomatoes, peanuts, and cotton.

112

Air pollution may be even more dangerous than experts have suspected. Studies reveal how tiny particles penetrate buildings and people's airways more quickly and deeply than previously known! We suggest you follow Bragg Super Power Breathing Exercises (pages 67-77) so you can improve your breathing of clean air to help offset damage from pollution and help improve your health and energy.

Your health is your true wealth. – Paul C. Bragg, N.D., Ph.D.

Polluted Air Becomes Polluted Water

Ammonia gas can contribute to *Eutrophication* – excessive growth of nutrients, from deposition or run-off, into natural waters, creeks, rivers, or lakes. *Eutrophication* causes a dense growth of plant life and death of animal life from lack of oxygen. Overgrowth of this choking algae vegetation or algal blooms disrupt normal functioning of the ecosystem, causing problems such as a lack of oxygen in the water, needed for fish and other aquatic life to survive! Water then becomes cloudy, colored a shade of green, yellow, or brown.

Smog Damages Buildings and Materials

The most visible characteristic of cities plagued with smog is the black and soot-covered windows, walls and other exposed surfaces! Yet, other damages can be seen. Sulfur dioxide corrodes metal and stone . . . damaging machinery and industrial instruments, as well as destroying buildings, statues, and monuments! Moreover, ground-level ozone has been found to bleach paints and coatings on buildings.

"CHEMTRAILS" – Toxic Heavy Metal Lead – Must Stop Being Sprayed into America's Skies

According to the EPA, a grand total of 571 tons of lead are dumped each year into the air from aircraft alone! The fuel that powers most propeller type aircraft, when burned is called "avgas." Tests show that avgas contains the following: Lead 48 ppm; Bromine 42.6 ppm and Chlorine 605.2 ppm. Lead is a highly toxic heavy metal that causes bone diseases, brain damage and cancer (more on lead bottom of page 104).

Avgas fuel is *emitting 86.4 kg of lead daily* into our air, and that lead falls onto our farming soils, forests, lakes, rivers, oceans and playgrounds. Avgas emissions are the number one source of lead emissions in the skies of America. Fortunately the FAA and EPA are teaming up to remove lead from avgas moving forward.

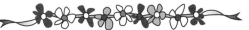

Airplanes are spraying chemicals across our skies that are on the OSHA hazardous list. Chemtrails show positive for toxic aluminum, barium, bacteria, virus, molds, causing health problems!

Do Know Air Quality Level in Your Area

Air quality is measured by a nationwide monitoring system that records concentrations of ozone and other pollutants. The EPA "translates" pollutant concentrations to a standard Air Quality Index (AQI). The higher the AQI value, the greater the danger! You may see the local AQI for ozone-smog reported in the weather section of your local newspaper, on television, or check web: *AirNow.gov.* Also if you have pollen allergies go to *Pollen. com* and enter your zip code to receive a 4-day allergen forecast for your area.

The Air Quaility Index (AQI)		
Ozone Concentration	AQI Values	Air Quality Description
0.0 to 0.064	0 to 50	Good
0.065 to 0.084	51 to 100	Moderate
0.085 to 0.104	101 to 150	Unhealthy for Sensitive Groups
0.105 to 0.124	151 to 200	Unhealthy

AQI by Color for Ozone & Particle Pollution

Green: is Good; index value 0-50; Air quality is satisfactory, and air pollution poses little or no risk.

Yellow: is Moderate; index value 51-100; Air quality is acceptable. However, there may be a risk for some people, particularly those who are unusually sensitive to air pollution.

Orange: is Unhealthy for Sensitive Groups; index value 101-150; Members of sensitive groups may experience health effects. The general public is less likely to be affected.

Red: is Unhealthy; index value 151-200; Some members of the general public may experience health effects; members of sensitive groups may experience more serious health effects.

Purple: is Very Unhealthy; index value 201-300; Health alert: The risk of health effects is increased for everyone.

Maroon: is Hazardous; index value 301 and higher; Health warning of emergency conditions: everyone is more likely to be affected. *(from AirNow.gov)*

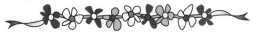

Average adult breathes over 3,000 gallons of air daily. – epa.gov/air

Healthful Solutions to Air Pollution

How can you supply your lungs, blood and whole body with clean healthy oxygen in this modern era of air pollution? **Oxygen, our invisible staff of life, is the greatest purifier and detoxifier, and is the body's basic life force.** First you must protect and strengthen your nose, sinuses, and your lungs, the first line of defense. Don't drink or eat any dairy products, for they increase mucus production and cause airway passages to swell! These conditions hinder your nose's ability to filter the air you breathe, which is needed to protect your lungs and health. Take care of your nose, sinuses and health! Work to develop powerful lungs that can withstand the challenges of polluted air when you're exposed to it.

Action 1   Do your Super Power Breathing Exercises in the early morning when air is cleaner and less contaminated.

Action 2   Regularly check air pollution levels in your area and plan accordingly. If you know your "Air Quality Index" (see chart page 114) is going to be high in your area, limit outdoor exercise.

Action 3   Avoid highly polluted areas during heavy smog.

115

Action 4   If you live in a smoggy area (*moving is best when possible*), **it's important to install the best HEPA air filters available** – particularly in rooms where you sleep, exercise and work; even have one in your car. Learn how to clean the filters and replace the pads so that they are always clean, washed and able to cleanse and purify the air. Move your room air purifier from room-to-room every six hours so the air in the entire house is cleaner.

Action 5   Keep indoor air as clean as possible! Don't smoke or be around smokers! Keep your house free of smoke, dust, and mold. Make sure fumes from gas stoves and heaters are properly vented! Reduce your use of chemical cleaners, insecticides, solvents and toxic paints.

––––––––––––––––––

Bring clean air into your home, office and car. Many people are unaware that exposure to indoor pollutants at home, at work and even new car vapors are often greater than levels found outdoors, causing serious health problems! Having an air purifier helps eliminate bacteria, viruses, mold, and other indoor pollutants. For more info on clean home air: Oreck.com and IQair.com

Action 6 Keep yourself healthy. Stop smoking. Eat well and exercise regularly. Fortify yourself internally with a multiple vitamin-mineral supplement, ample vitamin C and especially vitamin E (natural d-alpha mixed tocopherols), the body's oxygen protector. One of the vital functions of vitamin E is to regulate the use of oxygen by the body's cells. This helps assure that your life-giving oxygen is properly utilized for essential energy and that a reserve is retained in the red corpuscles for use when extra effort is needed. According to documented medical research, vitamin E helps increase the energy potential of all the oxygen you breathe by an amazing 25% to 50%! (see pages 151-153)

Action 7 Best to stay away from high traffic roads especially when on your daily brisk health walks.

Let's Clean-Up Our Air – For Our Health!

We can all help reduce ozone by taking the following steps:

- **Drive Less. Instead of a car, you may want to walk, use mass transit or ride a bike in safe bike lanes!**
- **Carpool/Rideshare when possible.**
- **Make sure your car is well-tuned.** Also take care not to over fill or spill gasoline when filling tank.
- **Make sure that you tightly seal** the lids of chemical products to keep the evaporation to a minimum.

Paving over land increases overall temperatures – and ozone forms more quickly at higher temperatures. More than one-half of commuting trips and 3 out of 4 shopping trips are less than 5 miles in length – perfect for cycling.

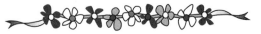

The more natural food you eat, the more you'll enjoy radiant health and be able to promote the higher life of love and brotherhood. – Patricia Bragg

Is there a relationship between breathing and diabetes, cancer, heart trouble, stress, asthma, emphysema, and other illnesses? YES! According to Framingham 30 year study that clarified breathing's direct relationship with longevity and the fact that many will lose 75% of their breathing capacity by age 75, if they don't take action and learn easy and safe ways to breathe better (web: breatheology.com). It's best to follow our Super Power Breathing Exercises (pages 67-77).

We Need the Protection of the Clean Air Act!

In many ways the problem of smog is worse now than 50 years ago. Hopefully we will never have air pollution disasters on the scale of some in the past. No one wants to live through suffering like that of the disastrous London smog attack of December 1952. A thermal inversion settled a fog on this great city on the Thames, trapping the pollutants spewed from its heavy industries and thousands of chimneys. Before the crisis abated, more than 12,000 people were dead and countless had fallen ill. Hospitals were inundated with patients suffering from *Cyanosis,* a condition in which a person actually turns blue for want of oxygen!

Today we fortunately have national and local agencies whose job is to prevent such past horrible smog disasters! These agencies constantly monitor air pollutant levels and atmospheric conditions. Based on their findings, guidelines and legislation is implemented to protect our health, but sadly problems do persist! The Environmental Protection Agency (EPA) notes that a larger number of Americans are living in areas that don't meet air quality standards. Too many urban areas don't meet federal standards of air quality – standards which are not safe enough to keep our air healthy! (*www.epa.gov*)

The EPA has approved more protective air quality standards. Studies show back in 2010 amendments from 1990 prevented 23,000 Americans from dying prematurely and averted over 1.7 million incidences of asthma attacks and aggravations of chronic asthma. In 2010 they prevented 67,000 incidences of chronic and acute bronchitis, 91,000 occurrences of shortness of breath, 4.1 million lost work days and 31 million days in which Americans would have had to restrict activity due to air pollution related illness! Because of new and improved safer standards, many cities and urban areas monitor air and are more alert to air pollution problems. We encourage you to become politically aware of all situations that affect your health in the area where you live! Vote for the laws and strong regulations that protect your health rights, especially to breathe clean, non-toxic air!

Clean energy laws generate new jobs and save consumers money. Transitioning to clean energy saves consumers billions on household energy costs. With the smart energy policies that promote a transition to renewable energy sources such as wind and sun, Americans benefit even more.

Clean Air Act Benefits and Costs

According to the EPA, the *benefits* of Clean Air Act programs have totaled trillions. Benefits involved a number of factors including – improved public health, avoided food crop damage, control of cancer-causing toxic air, the value of avoiding increases in illness and premature death, and the benefits to the ecosystem. If the Clean Air Act Amendments had not been enacted by 1990, 205,000 Americans would have died prematurely! Yes, millions more would have suffered from asthma and respiratory illnesses ranging from mild to severe!

Throughout the Clean Air Act, questions have been raised as to whether the health benefits of air pollution control justify the costs incurred by industry and taxpayers. The broader question is simple: How do the overall health, welfare, ecological and economic benefits of the *life-saving* Clean Air Act compare to these high cost programs? **The saving of human and animal health and food crops is reason enough to continue with programs to clean up the air we breathe and to protect lives and food crops!**

The results indicate that the benefits of the Clean Air Act and associated control programs substantially exceeded costs 30 to 1. A second important implication is that a large proportion of the cost benefits of Clean Air Act reductions comes in two major smog pollutants: lead and particulate matter. Not only monetarily, but from a health standpoint as well, **the Clean Air Act is vitally needed and important to our health and well-being!!!**

Negative factors like smog, soil and water pollutants, acid rain, UV radiation caused by the depletion of the earth's protective ozone layer, chemically treated foods, the disturbance of immune systems through repeated toxic vaccination and immunization, not to mention our stress-infused lifestyles, result in reduced immune response and the inability of our bodies to cope with or neutralize allergens. – Dr. Linda Page – Allergy Control & Management

We all grow healthier in nature, and with healthy foods, pure air, gentle sunshine and love!

My love of nature's beauty blesses me and gives me strength.
– Paul C. Bragg

Chapter 17

Doctor Natural Foods
Eating for Super Health, Energy and Longevity

Natural nutrition and correct breathing habits together will lift you to higher levels of vibration for happy, healthful living! To attain and maintain the peak of Super Health, we practice and recommend eating two balanced, healthy meals per day and taking a 24 to 32 hour distilled water cleansing fast each week. (Read pages 139, 142.)

Upon arising, before doing our Super Power Breathing Exercises, drink the apple cider vinegar drink: 2 tsps. of apple cider vinegar and raw honey (optional) in a glass of distilled water (see recipe on page 144).

After breathing exercises try to get some outdoor exercise: brisk walking, biking, swimming, hiking, weight-lifting, or gardening. Then have fresh fruit or the Bragg Health Energy Smoothie (recipe page 144) before getting busy with your days work.

119

We recommend your first real meal comes about mid-day. This gives the stomach a thorough rest of 16 to 18 hours, allowing it time to completely empty, recuperate and accumulate an abundant supply of new digestive juices after the previous evening's meal. Relax and chew each mouthful of food thoroughly *(remember your stomach has no teeth)* so the digestive process will have a good start and your food will be well assimilated to give you the health and energy needed!

Let food be your medicine and medicine be your food. Nature heals; the physician is only nature's assistant. – Hippocrates, 400 B.C.

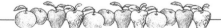

A healthy diet, along with apple cider vinegar and The Bragg Healthy Lifestyle will bring remarkable results. – "Woman's World Magazine"

Enjoy healthy, organic foods for their wonderful abundance of life energy.

The journey of a thousand miles begins with one step. – Lao Tzu

---

Now learn what great benefits a temperate diet will bring with it. In the first place, you will enjoy good health. – Horace, 65 B.C.

Power Salad for Lunch – Gives Energy & Health

A healthy, large salad of raw fruits or raw garden vegetables (organically grown is best) with raw nuts, sunflower or sesame seeds, soy or feta goats cheese for protein is an ideal delicious luncheon. Try our favorite Bragg Salad and Salad Dressing Recipes on page 145.

Most Americans have schedules which don't permit resting after the midday meal. But in Spain, Mexico and many countries worldwide, the main meal is at midday and is followed by a siesta. This short nap is ideal, giving you almost two fresh days in one! Rushed Americans eat their main meal in the evening and sadly millions eat a quick, unhealthy meal at fast food restaurants or in their car at noon.

Enjoy Healthy, Balanced Variety for Dinner

Relax at day's end with some Super Power Breaths. Cleanse the toxins from your lungs so that you will get the full benefit from a well-balanced, healthy nourishing and tasty dinner! Your basic health menu should include:

Salad: A smaller serving this time of fresh raw vegetables and salad greens or try one of these suggestions:

- Sliced red and green cabbage with diced red and green bell peppers and grated carrots
- grated carrots, sliced raw apples and raisins or try grated carrots, raisins, and diced pineapple
- lettuce, tomato, avocado and cucumber salad

Cooked Vegetables: Include green and yellow veggies; lightly cook, steam, bake, or stir-fry.

Protein Dish: Vegetable proteins include all beans, brown rice, lentils, tofu, etc., and raw, unsalted nuts and seeds. We recommend a vegetarian diet. If you do eat meat, limit it to 3 times a week and consider or try becoming a vegetarian. ***Never add table salt!*** Prepare your foods with healthy, nutritious flavors from fresh garlic, onions, and fresh herbs.

America badly needs to go on a healthy diet. We should do something about excessive, life-threatening fat. We should get rid of harmful obesity in the quickest possible way and this is by fasting (page 141). – Allan Cott, M.D.

Dessert: If desired, fresh organic fruits (apples, pears, etc.) are best when available, or unsweetened, stewed or dried fruit.

Beverages: For health, it's best not to drink beverages with meals, not even water! Your digestive juices do their best work undiluted! Have ample fluids one hour before and an hour after meals and during daytime. At least an hour after dinner, you may have the apple cider vinegar drink, some herbal tea or a glass of fresh fruit or vegetable juice. Drink all the distilled water you want between meals – ideal is eight glasses daily!

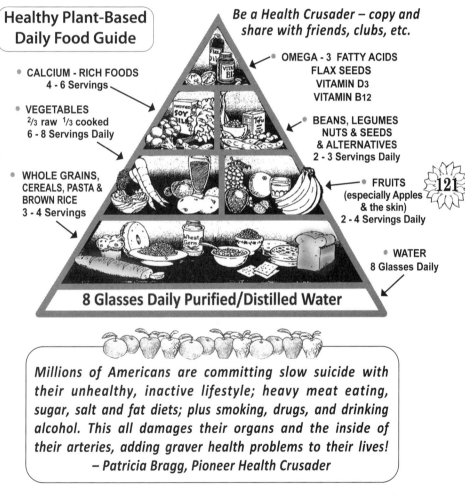

Healthy Plant-Based Daily Food Guide

Be a Health Crusader – copy and share with friends, clubs, etc.

* CALCIUM - RICH FOODS
  4 - 6 Servings

* VEGETABLES
  2/3 raw 1/3 cooked
  6 - 8 Servings Daily

* WHOLE GRAINS,
  CEREALS, PASTA &
  BROWN RICE
  3 - 4 Servings

* OMEGA - 3 FATTY ACIDS
  FLAX SEEDS
  VITAMIN D3
  VITAMIN B12

* BEANS, LEGUMES
  NUTS & SEEDS
  & ALTERNATIVES
  2 - 3 Servings Daily

* FRUITS
  (especially Apples
  & the skin)
  2 - 4 Servings Daily

* WATER
  8 Glasses Daily

121

8 Glasses Daily Purified/Distilled Water

Millions of Americans are committing slow suicide with their unhealthy, inactive lifestyle; heavy meat eating, sugar, salt and fat diets; plus smoking, drugs, and drinking alcohol. This all damages their organs and the inside of their arteries, adding graver health problems to their lives!
– Patricia Bragg, Pioneer Health Crusader

Eating apples can give you a burst of energy! Researchers found a significant boost in endurance capacity from quercetin in red apples. Quercetin (a phytonutrient – page 126) is a natural antioxidant that boosts the power of the mitochondria (the powerhouse of the cell) in muscles and the brain. This surge of power gives you energy!

Start Eating Healthy Foods For Super Energy

The *Healthy Plant-Based Daily Food Guide Pyramid* illustration (previous page) represents an ideal way of eating for achieving optimal nutrition, health and longevity! You will notice that this Food Guide Pyramid is based on healthy organic plant-based foods, with the emphasis on purified water, fruits, vegetables, whole grains, vegetable protein foods, non-dairy calcium foods, and raw nuts and seeds. This is the best diet for heart wellness, disease prevention and to enjoy longevity. *Eating a diet based on these dietary guidelines will help you get the nutrients needed for optimal health!*

•**Purified/Distilled Water:** This is the pyramid's foundation. We recommend *distilled water,* as it's the purest water for the body! Drink eight – 8 oz glasses of distilled water or pure, clean filtered water daily and even more if your lifestyle (sports and/or work) requires it.

•**Whole Grains:** Whole grains are pyramid's next level. Avoid all processed, refined GMO grain products and eat only unrefined, organic whole grain bread and cereal products! Grains such as quinoa, whole wheat, brown rice, barley, oats, millet, kamut, as well as 100% whole grain breads and cereals are best. One serving of whole grains is equal to 1 slice whole grain bread, 1 ounce ready-to-eat whole grain cereal, 1 cup cooked whole grains such as brown rice, oatmeal or other grains, 1 cup 100% whole wheat (or other whole grains) pasta or noodles, and 1 ounce of other whole grain products. We recommend eating 1-3 servings of organic, non-GMO whole grains daily.

•**Vegetables:** We recommend eating as many of your vegetables organic and raw (uncooked, in salads, juices, smoothies, etc.) as possible! When cooking vegetables, don't overcook them! Steaming or lightly stir-frying is best. The more colorful rainbow of vegetables you eat the better for your health as they contain more valuable healthful phytonutrients (see page 126). Eat a wide variety of organic vegetables daily. One vegetable serving is equal to 1 cup cooked vegetables or 1 cup raw uncooked vegetables, 1 cup salad, or 3/4 cup vegetable juice. We recommend having 6-8 or more vegetable servings daily.

- **Fruits:** Like vegetables, the more colorful the fruits the better they are for you. Enjoy organic fruits as much as possible! One serving of fruit is equal to 1 medium apple, banana, orange, pear or other fruit, $1/2$ cup fruit, $1/2$ cup of fruit juice or $1/4$ cup dried fruit. We recommend eating 4-6 servings or more of organic fruits daily.

- **Calcium-Rich Foods:** Are plant-derived calcium-rich foods. Plant sources of calcium are healthier than dairy products because they don't contain saturated fats or cholesterol. Healthy calcium-rich foods are: tofu, broccoli and green leafy vegetables. Examples of serving sizes of plant-derived calcium-rich foods include: $1/2$ cup tofu, $1/3$ cup almonds, 1 cup cooked or 2 cups high calcium dark greens (kale, collards, broccoli, bok choy or other Chinese greens), 1 cup calcium-rich beans (white, navy, Great Northern), $1/2$ cup seaweed, 1 tablespoon blackstrap molasses, 5 or more figs. We recommend having 4-6 servings of healthy non-dairy sources of calcium rich foods daily.

- **Beans, Legumes, Nuts & Seeds:** This group contains healthy protein foods. Vegetable protein foods are more optimal compared to animal protein foods. Vegetable proteins do not contain artery clogging saturated fats and cholesterol found in animal foods. They also contain protective factors to help prevent heart disease, cancer and diabetes. Vegetable proteins are high in quality and provide the body with the essential amino acids that it requires. One serving of vegetable protein foods include: 1 cup cooked legumes (beans, lentils, dried peas), $1/2$ cup firm tofu or tempeh, 1 serving of "veggie meat" alternate (e.g. veggie burger patty or soy patty), 3 tablespoons nut or seed butter, 1 cup soy milk. We recommend you have 2 to 3 or more vegetable protein servings daily with meals.

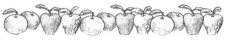

Life cannot be maintained unless life be taken in. And this is best done by making at least 60% of your diet raw and with a plentiful supply of fresh juicy organic fruits and some lightly cooked vegetables. – Patricia Bragg

---

Grains that are heart-healthy are organic brown rice, organic whole grain breads, cereals, and pastas. There's also buckwheat, barley, millet, and tasty quinoa is a complete protein and makes an ideal breakfast cereal. Also popcorn, organic corn is a whole grain.

•Healthy Fats, Essential Fatty Acids, Omega-3 and Other Nutrients: Servings of healthy fats include: 1 tsp. flaxseed oil (flaxseed is high in phytonutrients called lignans), 1 Tbsp of extra-virgin olive oil, 3 tsps. raw walnuts. Be sure to provide your body with the nutritional supplements your body requires for optimal health (page 174).

What are Nature's Miracle Phytonutrients?

These wonderful, organic compounds are found in plants, ('phyto' means 'plant' in Greek), that are vital to human health. Increasingly, scientific studies are showing that phytonutrients help protect us from many serious health issues, including heart disease and stroke. Organic fruits, vegetables, grains, legumes, nuts, seeds and some teas are rich in the miracle phytonutrients.

Physicians and Scientists have written about the critical nature of these foods for thousands of years, but the specific benefits of phytonutrients are still being discovered. They are created when plants absorb energy from the earth, water, air and sun. This energy helps plants survive environmental challenges such as diseases, injures, drought, excessive heat, ultraviolet sunrays and poisons. This incredible energy forms an important part of the plant's immune system! It appears to provide humans with the same benefits, when we consume the plants! They help increase our immune and regeneration systems. **Plants give us strength, endurance, health and ultimately help us feel better and live longer.**

To Make Organic Nut Butters:

Grind 1 1/2 cups of raw unsalted organic nuts in a food processor or blender. Continue grinding nuts down until they are a thick, fudge-like paste. Then add sunflower or nut oil (start with 1 Tbsp and add more only if necessary), blend until smooth. Best kept refrigerated.

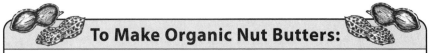

Chia Seeds: (Bragg promoted in 1940) – are rich in omega-3 fatty acids and antioxidants! Chia seeds provide fiber and calcium, phosphorus, magnesium, iron, niacin and zinc. They help slow down how fast our bodies convert carbohydrates into simple sugars, which may have great benefits for diabetics.

Antioxidant & Phytonutrient Health Benefits

The body must have these phytonutrients and enzymes to break food down, kill viruses and bacteria and dissolve tumors! A diet of at least 50% raw, unprocessed foods is vital to make sure that we are getting enough enzymes and phytonutrients to optimize the body's processes.

Plants contain more than 10,000 phytonutrients, one reason 10-14 servings of fruits and veggies daily are recommended. Plants and vegetables contain different phytonutrients, so having a variety in your diet is important.

On average, plant foods have 64 times more antioxidants than animal foods, which is critical because when it comes to antioxidants, the more we eat, the more our health benefits! **Eating a diet high in antioxidants is important because they reduce inflammation and free radicals in the body** and help protect against heart disease and cancer. See chart page 126 for health benefits of different plant sources.
See: *hsph.Harvard.edu/NutritionSource/antioxidants*.

Main Sources of Miracle Phytonutrients

The following are high in phytonutrients: carrots and yellow vegetables (sweet potatoes and pumpkins), peaches, apricots, broccoli, leafy greens (kale, spinach, turnip greens), tomatoes, pink grapefruit, watermelon, guava, blackberries, walnuts, strawberries, cranberries, raspberries, blueberries, grape juice, prunes, red cabbage, pineapple, oranges, plums, pinto beans, spinach, kiwi fruit and red peppers.

The more live, unprocessed foods we eat the more phytonutrients and enzymes we consume the healthier our diet. This natural food is full of energy we need to live longer, healthier lives! To boost your immune system and cell regeneration eat more phytonutrients, practice deep breathing exercises daily, get physical exercise, and make sure your diet is at least 50% raw, healthy, organic foods! That's The Bragg Healthy Lifestyle and when followed it produces miracles.

Increasing intake of fruits and vegetables can help you prevent heart disease, cancer and other chronic diseases. Surveys show those who increased their daily fruit and vegetable intake improved their health, vitality and well-being.
– UC Berkeley Wellness Letter • www.BerkeleyWellness.com

Mother Nature's Miracle Phytonutrients Help Prevent Cancer:

Make sure to get your daily dose of naturally occurring, cancer-fighting super foods – Phytonutrients are abundant in apples, tomatoes, onions, garlic, beans, legumes, soybeans, cabbage, cauliflower, broccoli, citrus, etc. Champions with highest count of Phytonutrients – apples and tomatoes.

Phytonutrient	Food Sources	Health Action
PHYTOESTROGEN ISOFLAVONES	Soy products, flaxseed, seeds and nuts, yams, alfalfa, pomegranates lentils, carrots, apples	Helps block some cancers, aids in menopausal symptoms, balances hormones, helps improve memory, enhances heart health
PHYTOSTEROLS	Plant oils: corn, sesame, safflower; rice bran, wheat germ, peanuts	Blocks hormonal role in cancers, inhibits uptake of cholesterol from diet, reduce risk of heart attack
LIGNANS	Flaxseeds, rye, lentils, soy mushrooms, barley	Helps prevent breast cancer, heart disease and balances hormones
SAPONINS	Yams, beets, beans, cabbage, nuts, soybeans	Helps prevent cancer cells from multiplying, reduces cholesterol
TERPENES	Carrots, winter squash, sweet potatoes, yams, apples, cantaloupes, cherries	Antioxidants – protects DNA from free radical-induced damage, and improves immunity
	Tomatoes and its sauces, tomato-based products	Helps block UVA & UVB and offers help to protect against cancers – breast, prostate, etc.
	Spinach, kale, beet and turnip greens, cabbage	Protects eyes from macular degeneration,
	Red chile peppers	Keeps carcinogens from binding to DNA
QUERCETIN (& FLAVONOIDS)	Apples (especially the skins), red onions and green tea	Strong cancer fighter, protects heart - arteries. Reduces pain, allergy and asthma symptoms
	Citrus fruits (flavonoids)	Promotes protective enzymes
PHENOLS	Apples, fennel, parsley, carrots, alfalfa, cabbage	Helps prevent blood clotting & has important anticancer properties
	Cinnamon	Promotes healthy blood sugar and glucose metabolism
	Citrus fruits, broccoli, cabbage, cucumbers, green peppers, tomatoes	Antioxidants – flavonoids, block membrane receptor sites for certain hormones
	Apples, grape seeds	Strong antioxidants; fights germs and bacteria, strengthens immune system, veins and capillaries
	Grapes, especially skins	Antioxidant, antimutagen; promotes detoxification. Acts as carcinogen inhibitors
	Yellow and green squash	Antihepatotoxic, antitumor
SULFUR COMPOUNDS	Onions and garlic, (fresh is always best) Red onions (our favorite) also contain Quercetin Onions help keep doctor away	Promotes liver enzymes, inhibits cholesterol synthesis, reduces triglycerides, lowers blood pressure improves immune response, fights infections, germs and parasites

The Bragg Healthy Lifestyle Promotes Super Health and Super Energy!

When you eat according to The Bragg Healthy Lifestyle, 60% to 70% of your diet will consist of fresh, raw, live foods (organic is best): Raw veggies, salads, fresh fruits and juices, sprouts, raw seeds and nuts. Enjoy 100% whole grain breads (home-baked is best), whole grain pastas and cereals, organic brown rice, beans and legumes. You can make healthy and delicious combination salads, soups, casseroles, etc., and the nutritious blender drinks that all ages will love. These are the healthy, no cholesterol, low-sodium live foods which provide good body fuel for more increased health and vitality. **These wholesome foods make joyous, healthy, energized people!**

Following The Bragg Healthy Lifestyle, you will become revitalized and reborn into a fresh new life filled with joy, vitality, youthfulness and longevity! There are millions of healthy Bragg followers around the world who have proven to themselves that this Healthy Lifestyle works miracles when followed faithfully. **For more info on the lifestyle that keeps you ageless, read the book *Bragg Healthy Lifestyle – Vital Living at Any Age*** (See back pages for Bragg book list).

127

Bad Nutrition – #1 Cause of Sickness

"Diet-related diseases account for 68% of all deaths."
– Dr. C. Everett Koop

America's former Surgeon General and our friend, said this in his famous 1988 landmark report on nutrition and health in America. People don't die of infectious conditions as such,

Dr. Koop & Patricia
Hawaii Health Conference

but of malnutrition that allows the germs to get a foothold in sickly bodies! Also, bad nutrition is usually the cause of non-infectious, fatal or degenerative conditions. When the body has its full nutrition quota of vitamin and minerals, including potassium, it's almost impossible for germs to get a foothold in a healthy, powerful bloodstream and tissues!

Former U.S. Surgeon General, Dr. C. Everett Koop said –
"Paul Bragg did more for the Health of America than any one person I know."

Eliminating Meat is Safer and Healthier

Play it safe, become a healthy vegetarian! Commercial cattle are fed antibiotics, growth hormones and dead, ground up carcasses of other feed lot animals who didn't make it to the slaughterhouse. If you eat meat or poultry, buy organic/hormone and antibiotic free. See informative web: *www.EarthSave.org*.

Meat is also a major source of toxic uric acid and cholesterol, both harmful to your health. If you are going to include meat in your diet, it should not be eaten more than 2 times a week. In our opinion, fresh fish can be the least toxic of the flesh proteins. But beware of fish from polluted waters! They can be loaded with mercury, lead, cadmium, DDT and many other toxic substances. If you are unable to test the waters from where your fish come, don't risk eating them! And avoid shellfish – shrimp, lobster and crayfish. They are garbage-eating bottom-feeders – the rats and flies of the water kingdom. They eat all of the rotting, decaying scum and refuse off the bottoms of the oceans, lakes and rivers. Next come chicken and turkey (never eat the skin, which is heavy in cholesterol). Third place goes to lamb and beef.

128

People should not eat pork or pork products. The pig is the only animal besides man that develops arteriosclerosis or hardening of the arteries. In fact, this animal is so loaded with cholesterol that in cold weather, unprotected pigs and hogs will become solid and stiff, as though frozen solid. Also, this animal is often infected with a dangerous parasite which causes trichinosis.

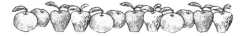

Scientists agree that bacon, sausage and other processed meats and red meats cause cancer. A World Health Organization study suggests that an additional 3.5 oz. of red meat everyday raises risk of colorectal cancer by 17%; eating an additional 1.8 oz. of processed meat daily raises risk by 18%. About 34,000 cancer deaths a year worldwide are attributable to diets high in processed meats. Red meat includes beef, veal, pork, lamb, mutton and goat. Processed meat includes hot dogs, ham, sausages, corned beef and jerky.

The secret of longevity is eating intelligently healthy. – Gaylord Hauser

Plant-Based Protein Chart

BEANS & LEGUMES

(1 cup cooked)	PROTEIN IN GRAMS
Soybeans	29
Lentils	18
Adzuki Beans	17
Cannellini	17
Navy Beans	16
Split Peas	16
Black Beans	15
Garbanzos (chick peas)	15
Kidney Beans	15
Great Northern Beans	15
Lima Beans	15
Black-eyed Peas	14
Pinto Beans	14
Mung Beans	14
Tofu (3 oz.)	7 to 12
Green Peas (whole)	9

RAW NUTS & SEEDS

(1/4 cup or 4 Tbsps)	PROTEIN IN GRAMS
Chia Seeds	12
Macadamia Nuts	11
Flax Seeds	8
Sunflower Seeds	8
Almonds	7
Pumpkin Seeds	7
Sesame Seeds	7
Walnuts	5
Brazil Nuts	5
Hazelnuts	5
Pine Nuts	4
Cashews	4

NUT BUTTERS

(2 Tbsps)	PROTEIN IN GRAMS
Peanut Butter	7 to 9
Almond Butter	5 to 8
Cashew Butter	4 to 5
Sesame - Tahini	6

VEGETABLES

(1 Serving or 1 cup)	PROTEIN IN GRAMS
Spirulina	8.6
Corn (1 cob)	5
Potato (with skin)	5
Mushrooms, Oyster	5
Artichoke (1 medium)	4
Collard Greens	4
Broccoli	4
Brussel Sprouts	4
Mushrooms, Shitake	3.5
Swiss Chard	3
Kale	2.5
Asparagus (5 spears)	2
String Beans	2
Beets	2
Peas	2
Sweet Potato	3
Summer Squash	2
Cabbage	2
Carrot	2
Cauliflower	2
Squash	2
Celery	1
Spinach	1
Bell Peppers	1
Cucumber	1
Eggplant	1
Leeks	1
Lettuce	1
Tomato (1 medium)	1
Radish	1
Turnips	1

DAIRY & NUT MILKS

(1 cup)	PROTEIN IN GRAMS
Oat Milk	3 to 4
Almond Milk	1 to 2
Rice Milk	1
Eggs (1) *(free-range)*	6

FRUITS

(1 Serving or 1 cup)	PROTEIN IN GRAMS
Avocado (1 medium)	4
Banana (1)	1 to 2
Blackberries (1 cup)	2
Pomegranate (1)	1.5
Blueberries (1 cup)	1
Cantaloupe (1 cup)	1
Cherries (1 cup)	1
Grapes (1 cup)	1
Honeydew (1 cup)	1
Kiwi (1 large)	1
Lemon (1)	1
Mango (1)	1
Nectarine (1)	1
Orange (1)	1
Peach (1)	1
Pear (1)	1
Pineapple (1 cup)	1
Plum (1)	1
Raspberries (1 cup)	1
Strawberries (1 cup)	1
Watermelon (1 cup)	1

129

GRAINS & RICE

(1 cup cooked)	PROTEIN IN GRAMS
Triticale	25
Millet	8.4
Kamut	11
Amaranth	7
Oat Bran	7
Wild Rice	7
Couscous (whole wheat)	6
Bulgar Wheat	6
Buckwheat	6
Teff	6
Oat Groats	6
Barley	5
Quinoa	5
Brown Rice	5
Spelt	5

This chart displays the protein content of common vegetarian foods.
Note that in order to determine the amount of protein that is optimal for your body, use the following formula that is based on a vegan diet: *the RDA recommends that we take in 0.36 grams of protein per pound that we weigh* (100 lbs. x 0.36 = 36 grams).

Unhealthy Diet Depletes Minerals in Body

Unbalanced and unhealthy diets can deplete the body of calcium, magnesium, potassium and other major elements (page 154). Diets high in proteins, meats, fish, and eggs may provide excess phosphorus which depletes calcium and magnesium from bones and tissues. This causes these minerals to be lost in the urine. High fat diets tend to increase the uptake of phosphorus from the intestines relative to calcium and other basic minerals. High phosphorus diet sodas can also produce losses of calcium and magnesium.

Deficiencies of calcium and magnesium can produce many different health problems, from osteoporosis to muscular cramping, hyperactivity, muscular twitching (Restless Leg Syndrome effects millions), sleep disorders and frequency of urination. Deficiencies or imbalances of other minerals can produce many other health problems.

It is very important to clean and detoxify the body through fasting and by drinking 8 glasses of pure distilled water and organically grown vegetable and fruit juices. In order to continually provide the body with new supplies of minerals, adults need a diet containing a variety of organic vegetables, as well as mineral rich kelp and other sea vegetables. Infants, also need healthy mother's milk, preferably to one year of age and longer when possible for a solid foundation to grow from!

Many adults and children in western civilizations are malnourished and have low levels of essential minerals in their bodies due to losses from consuming coffee, tea, cola and carbonated beverages and processed foods and unhealthy diets containing refined flours, sugar and salt.

The body's organ systems can become so unbalanced by chronic stress; from toxins in our air, water and soil; by disease-produced injuries; and in babies, by prenatal nutritional deficiencies in the mother's diet and their unhealthy lifestyle habits! Thus, people in our fast-food society wisely need natural multi-vitamin and mineral food supplements to ensure they get their vital nutrients. We suggest everyone take them for extra protection.

"Sickness is a Crime – Don't Be a Criminal."

Do Not Poison Your Body with Unhealthy, Toxic, Foodless Foods and Harmful Drinks!

In our industrialized, urbanized civilization, we pay a heavy price for the convenience of mass distribution of foodstuffs. Not only has our flour been bleached and robbed of its vital wheat germ, but the majority of commercial foods have been devitalized, demineralized – rendered foodless – in order to give them a longer shelf life! You are risking your own life when you eat these foodless foods that cannot nourish your body properly! Many contain preservatives and additives (such as nitrates and nitrites) whose cumulative effect has proven to be extremely harmful to the human body.

Even though the Federal Food & Drug Administration (FDA) requires label listing of ingredients on processed, packaged and canned foods, few people bother to read the label's fine print. If they do, they rarely understand it or take the trouble to find out what the various additives are and what effect they have on the human body! You don't have to be a chemist to find answers; just *Google* and become educated.

131

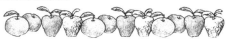

I live on legumes, vegetables and fruits. No dairy, no meat of any kind, no chicken, no turkey, and very little fish, once in a while. It changed my metabolism and I lost 24 pounds. I did research and found 82% of people who go on a plant-based diet begin to heal themselves, as I did.
– U.S. President Bill Clinton, 1993-2001

Love, kindness and compassion are necessities, not luxuries . . . without them humanity cannot survive. – The Dalai Lama

We love helping people who want to live and follow The Bragg Healthy Lifestyle! We want to help you now!

HEALTHY SNACK MUNCHING: Teenagers do a lot of their snacking and eating away from home, buying food from theaters, vending machines, fast-food outlets, shopping mall food courts, etc. But when armed with the right health guidance from parents and healthy school food programs, they can wisely select and be satisfied with healthy choices: fruits and juice drinks, whole grain and honey bakery items rather than high-fat, sugared, white flour snacks that are mostly void of nutrition, and harmful to health, plus can cause weight gain, diabetes and obesity.

For example, *Webster's Dictionary* defines **nitrate** as a *"salt or ester of nitric acid"* and defines **nitric acid** as a *"corrosive liquid inorganic acid HN0₃."* Ordinary common sense can figure out what a steady diet of toxic foods containing a concentrated form of a corrosive liquid inorganic acid will do to your body! **Nitrates and nitrites are deadly preservatives. Avoid them like the plague!**

Sulphur dioxide is another commercial preservative commonly used on dried fruits. It is defined by Webster as a *"heavy pungent gas, easily condensed to a colorless liquid and used especially in making sulfuric acid."* Do we have to remind you that sulfuric acid eats away flesh?

Many natural fats and oils are ruined by *hydrogenation*. This toxic hardening process keeps them from becoming rancid, but renders them absolutely indigestible and can cause terrible clogging of the cardiovascular system. Read all labels and understand them! Stop eating all commercially refined and processed foods made with refined white flour, refined white sugar, processed lunch meats and cheeses and foods with hydrogenated fats, harmful additives and preservatives such as sodium nitrate, MSG (monosodium glutamate), and sulfur dioxide.

Also avoid soft drinks and cola drinks! They contain toxic fluoridated water, artificial flavors, colors, preservatives and sweeteners. They will slowly poison your bloodstream and body. The huge quantities of phosphorus in soda depletes calcium and magnesium from the body. Result: millions suffer with osteoporosis.

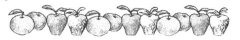

Just one caffeinated drink – a soft drink, caffeinated tea or coffee, will put your body on the caffeine roller-coaster. Caffeine doesn't provide energy to your system, it just burns up your reserves faster. You get a short-term boost at the expense of long-term jitters and fatigue. When an adrenal coffee high wears off, you feel the drop in terms of fatigue, irritability, mood swings, depression, headache or confusion.
– Stephen Cherniske, author "Caffeine Blues"

The Bragg Healthy Lifestyle helps make a healthier you and a healthier world!

Avoid These Processed, Refined, Harmful Foods:

Once you realize the harm caused to your body by unhealthy refined, chemicalized, deficient foods, you'll want to eliminate "killer" foods:

- **Refined sugar / artificial sweeteners** (toxic aspartame) or their products such as jams, jellies, preserves, marmalades, yogurts, ice cream, sherbets, Jello, cake, candy, cookies, all chewing gum, colas and diet drinks, pies, pastries, and all sugared fruit juices and fruits canned in sugar syrup. (Health Stores have delicious healthy replacements, such as Stevia, raw honey, 100% maple syrup, and agave nectar, so seek and buy the best).

- **White flour products** such as white bread, wheat-white bread, enriched flours, rye bread that has white flour in it, dumplings, biscuits, buns, gravy, pasta, pancakes, waffles, soda crackers, pizza, ravioli, pies, pastries, cakes, cookies, prepared and commercial puddings and ready-mix bakery products. Most are made with dangerous (oxy-cholesterol) powdered milk and powdered eggs. (Health Stores have a variety of 100% non-GMO whole grain organic products, breads, chips, crackers, pastas, desserts).

- **Salted foods**, such as pretzels, corn chips, potato chips, crackers and nuts.

- **Refined white rice** and pearl barley. • **Fried fast foods**. • **Indian ghee**.

- **Refined dry processed cereals** that are sugared, such as cornflakes, etc.

- **Foods that contain Olestra**, palm and cottonseed oil.

- **Peanuts and peanut butter** that contain hydrogenated, hardened oils and any peanuts with mold and all molds that can cause allergies.

- **Margarine** – combines heart-deadly trans-fatty acids and saturated fats.

- **Saturated fats and hydrogenated oils** – enemies that clog the arteries.

- **Coffee, soft drinks, teas, alcohol, sugared juices** – even if decaffeinated.

- **Fresh pork / products.** • **Fried, fatty, greasy meats.** • **Irradiated GMO foods**.

- **Smoked meats**, such as ham, bacon, sausage and all smoked fish.

- **Luncheon meats**, hot dogs, salami, bologna, corned beef, pastrami and packaged meats containing dangerous sodium nitrate or nitrite.

- **Dried fruits** containing sulphur dioxide – a toxic preservative.

- **Chickens, turkeys and meats injected with hormones** or fed with commercial feed containing any drugs or toxins.

- **Canned soups** – read labels for sugar, salt, starch, flour and preservatives.

- **Foods containing preservatives, additives**, benzoate of soda, salt, sugar, cream of tartar, drugs, irradiated and genetically engineered foods.

- **Day-old cooked vegetables**, potatoes and pre-mixed, wilted lifeless salads.

- **All commercial vinegars:** pasteurized, filtered, distilled, white, malt and synthetic vinegars are dead vinegars! (We use only unfiltered Apple Cider Vinegar with "Mother Enzyme" as used in olden times.)

Please follow The Bragg Healthy Lifestyle to provide the basic, healthy nourishment to maintain your precious health.

133

Modern GMO Wheat –
No Longer Mother Nature's Wheat!!!

Modern GMO wheat isn't really the wheat that Mother Nature intended. About 700 million tons of wheat are grown worldwide making it second most-produced grain after corn. It's grown on more land area than any other commercial crop and considered a staple food for humans.

The Wheat We Eat Today Isn't
the Wheat Our Grandmothers Ate!

The balance and ratio of nutrients that "Mother Nature" created for wheat has been modified! At some point in our history, this ancient grain was nutritious, however modern GMO wheat really isn't the same wheat at all. Once agribusiness took over to develop a higher-yielding crop, wheat became hybridized to the extent it has completely transformed from its prehistorical genetic configuration.

The majority of wheat is processed into 60% extraction or bleached white flour. The standard for most wheat products means that 40% of the original wheat grain is removed! So not only do we have an unhealthier, modified, and hybridized strain of wheat, we also remove and further degrade its nutritional value by processing it!

Unfortunately, the 40% that gets removed includes the bran and the germ of the wheat grain – its most nutrient-rich parts. In the process of making 60% extraction flour, most of the vitamin B1, B2, B3, E, folic acid, calcium, phosphorus, zinc, copper, iron, and fiber sadly are lost. **Any processed foods with GMO wheat are unhealthy since they cause more body health risks than benefits.**

Heavily marketed white carbs (white sugar, flour, pasta, etc.) that are packaged in boxes are designed to make you crave more. They're not good for your body, your mind or your soul!

Seek out, and choose healthy whole foods: organic fruits, vegetables, rice, beans, nuts, seeds, etc. rather than commercial, refined white flour and sugar products and highly processed canned goods in center aisles.

People who turn away from GMO wheat have dropped substantial weight. Even diabetics no longer become diabetic; people with arthritis have dramatic relief; and less acid reflux; leg swelling; and irritable bowel syndrome.

"The whiter the bread, the sooner you're dead!" The body doesn't recognize processed GMO wheat as food. Nutrient absorption from processed wheat products is thus consequential with almost no nutritional value.

Even if you choose 100% whole wheat products they are based on modern GMO wheat strains created by irradiation of wheat seeds and embryos with chemicals, gamma rays, and high-dose X-rays to induce mutations. You are still consuming genetically modified grain.

To avoid all the toxic GMO wheat-oriented products, eat healthy foods – organic nuts, fruits and vegetables along with products made with non-GMO organic grains.

Health Problems Associated With GMO Wheat

Dr. Marcia Alvarez who specializes in nutritional programs for obese patients says, **"Modern GMO wheat grains could certainly be considered as the root of all evil in the world of nutrition** since they cause so many documented health problems across so many populations in the world." *www.NonGMOproject.org*

Dr. Alvarez asserted that modern GMO wheat is now responsible for more intolerances than almost any other food in the world! "In my practice of over two decades, we have documented that for every ten people with digestive problems, obesity, irritable bowel syndrome, diabetes, arthritis and even heart disease, 8 out of 10 people have health problems with wheat! Once we remove modern GMO wheat from their diets, most of their symptoms disappear within 3 to 6 months," she added. Dr. Alvarez estimates that between the influx of genetically modified (GMO) strains of wheat and current growing tendencies of wheat elimination worldwide, a trend is emerging in the next 20 years that will likely see 80% of people stop their consumption of GMO wheat in any form!

If you select 100% organic whole wheat products, the bran and germ of the wheat will remain in the product, and the health benefits will be impressive! Organic non-GMO whole wheat is a good dietary fiber source.

Food fiber is vital for good health, healthy elimination and adequate intake helps prevent colon cancer! Everyone should benefit from making sure they regularly include foods in their diet such as organic non-GMO whole grains, barley, oats, beans, fruits and vegetables that provide healthy food fibers.

Caution Using Salt – It's a Slow Killer!

We can't stress it enough: Avoid using salt!

The *salt of the earth* (inorganic sodium chloride) is poisonous to humans, plants and animals. What about *salt licks?* Don't even wild animals crave salt? My father investigated this thoroughly – and found that salt licks never contain sodium chloride. They are decomposed plant life made into organic minerals. Commercial salt licks used by cattle ranchers are to make cattle thirsty so they will drink volumes of water (like bars offering free pretzels). Cattle weighing more (means more money) when the time comes for them to be sold. This is why meat *shrinks* excessively when cooked.

Salt was the first food preservative discovered by man. Remember, they had no refrigeration or means of storing food for long periods. Because their lifestyles were extremely active, their bodies could eliminate this indigestible salt, an inorganic mineral that plays havoc in the body. They stayed healthy until introduced to western diet poisons! Then their deterioration was rapid and tragic. My father and I have seen this especially in the South Sea islands, Hawaii, Samoa and Tahiti!

Most civilized people over 40 today are sedentary creatures. Most cannot eliminate or assimilate the excessive amount of salt they eat. Their bodies stash it away in crystals that harden in the artery lining and blood vessels and in joints, feet and hands, causing arthritis and pain! Some salt is stored in a water solution that bloats the tissues. This can cause congestive heart failure and even death. Eliminate table salt from your diet! Achieve marvelous flavors by a skillful use of herbs, garlic, onions and mushrooms. Also apple cider vinegar and lemon juice are good seasoners for salads, veggies, beans, rice, and legumes.

Refined salt actually deadens your taste buds. Stay away from refined salt – we do! Your taste buds will awaken and soon start to enjoy the natural flavors of foods you eat. Even more importantly, you will become healthier and live longer when you give up salt and live a 100% healthy lifestyle!

Avoid health-destroying habits: sugar, fat, salt, refined foods and refined flours, chemical preservatives, soda and alcohol.

8 Glasses Pure Water – Essential for Health!

Distilled water is the world's purest and best water! It's excellent for detoxification and fasting programs because it helps cleanse and flush toxins and harmful substances out of the body cells, organs and fluids of the body! Pure, clean filtered water from a reliable water company, reverse osmosis system or alkaline water system is also safe to drink.

Most water from chemically-treated public water systems, and even some wells and springs, likely contains harmful chemicals and toxic elements (toxic fluorides, chlorides, etc.). Too often the water in our homes, offices, schools, and public buildings can be loaded with toxins; zinc, copper, cadmium or even lead from old soldered pipes.

The pure water from the fresh juices of vegetables and fruits, or the clean rain (distilled) water or steam (bottled) distilled water is essential for super health! Your body is constantly working for you. Your body is 75% water. The liquids you put in it will either nourish you or harm you, and may even eventually kill you!

Your body constantly breaks down old bone and tissue cells and replaces them with new ones! As your body casts off old minerals and broken-down cells, it must obtain new supplies of essential elements in order to make healthy, new cells! (Important reason to eat healthy foods.)

Scientists discovered that many disorders, including dental problems, different types of arthritis, osteoporosis and some forms of hardening of the arteries are in part due to imbalances in the levels and ratios of minerals in the body. Every body requires a proper balance of all the nutritive elements in order to remain healthy. It's as bad for a person to have too much of one item as it is to have too little of another. In order for calcium to be able to create new cells of bone and teeth, you must have adequate levels of phosphorus and magnesium. Yet, if there is too much of these minerals or too little calcium, etc. in the diet, old bone will be taken away, however new bone will not be formed. Read more info page 154.

THE 75% WATERY HUMAN

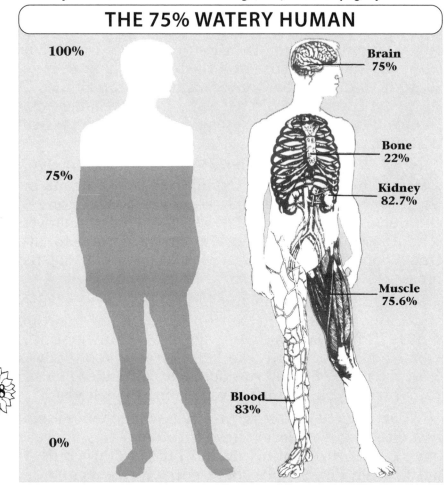

100%

75%

0%

Brain
75%

Bone
22%

Kidney
82.7%

Muscle
75.6%

Blood
83%

138

The amount of water in the body, averaging 75%, varies considerably and even from one part of the body to another area (illustration on right). A lean man may hold 75% of his weight in body water, while a woman – because of her larger proportion of water-poor fatty tissues – may be only 52% water. The lowering of water content in the blood is what triggers the hypothalamus, the brain's vital thirst center, to send out its familiar urgent demand for a drink of water! Please obey and drink ample amounts of purified water. By the time you feel thirsty, you're already dehydrated.
– American Running and Fitness Association

Water Percentage in Various Body Parts:

Teeth	10%	Spleen	75.5%
Bones	22%	Lungs	80%
Cartilage	55%	Blood	83%
Red blood corpuscles	68.7%	Bile	86%
Liver	71.5%	Plasma	90%
Brain	75%	Lymph	94%
Muscle tissue	75%	Saliva	95.5%

This chart shows why 8-10 glasses of pure water daily are so important.

Juice Fast – Introduction to Water Fast

Fasting has been rediscovered, through juice fasting, as a simple, easy means of cleansing and restoring health and vitality. To fast (*abstain from food, not water*) comes from an Old English word *fasten* or *to hold firm*. It's a means to commit oneself to the task of finding inner strength through body, mind and soul cleansing. Throughout history the world's greatest philosophers and sages – including Socrates, Plato, Buddha, Gandhi and Jesus – practiced fasting and preached its great physical and spiritual benefits!

Juice bars are springing up everywhere and juice fasting has become very popular. Those who believe in the power and effectiveness of juice and water fasting say fasting helps balance their lives physically, mentally, spiritually and emotionally. Although we feel a water fast is best, an introductory liquid juice fast can offer people an ideal opportunity to give their intestinal systems a restful, cleansing relief from the high fat, high sugar, high salt and high protein fast foods that so many Americans unhealthily exist on!

Organic, raw, live fruit and vegetable juices can be purchased fresh from Health Stores, farmer's markets and many super markets. You can also prepare healthy juices yourself using a home juicer. When juice fasting, it's best to dilute juice with $1/3$ distilled water. The list on next page gives you many delicious combination ideas.

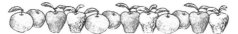

Fasting is an effective and safe method of detoxifying the body
– a healing technique used for centuries. Fasting regularly
one day a week can help the body cleanse and heal itself.
Bragg Books were my conversion to the healthy way.
– James Balch, M.D. co-author of "Prescription for Nutritional Healing"

The three greatest letters in the English alphabet are N-O-W.
There is no time like the present. Begin Now!
– Sir Walter Scott, Scottish Poet

Organic whole grains, vegetables, fruits, raw nuts and seeds give needed
vitamins and minerals to the body. – Patricia Bragg, Health Crusader

Here are Some Powerful Juice Combinations:

1. Beet, celery, kale and carrots
2. Cabbage, celery and apple
3. Cabbage, cucumber, celery, tomato, kale, spinach and basil
4. Tomato, carrot and celery
5. Carrot, celery, kale garlic, watercress, blue or goji berries and wheatgrass
6. Grapefruit, orange and lemon
7. Beet, parsley, celery, carrot, mustard greens, cabbage, garlic
8. Beet, celery, kale and carrot
9. Cucumber, carrot and parsley
10. Watercress, apple, cucumber, garlic
11. Asparagus, carrot and apple
12. Carrot, celery, kale, parsley and cabbage, onion, sweet basil
13. Carrot, coconut milk and ginger
14. Carrot, broccoli, lemon, cayenne
15. Carrot, sprouts, kelp, rosemary
16. Apple, carrot, radish, ginger
17. Apple, pineapple and seaweed
18. Apple, papaya and grapes
19. Papaya, blueberries and apple
20. Leafy greens, broccoli, apple
21. Grape, apple and blueberries
22. Watermelon (best alone)

Paul C. Bragg Introduced Juicing to America

Juicing has come a long way since the first hand operated vegetable-fruit juicers were available. Before, this juice was pressed by hand using cheesecloth. He introduced his new juice therapy idea, then pineapple juice, then later tomato juice, to the American public. These two juices were erroneously thought to be too acidic! Now, these health beverages have become the favorites of millions. TV's famous Juicemen Jack LaLanne and Jay Kordich say Paul Bragg was their early inspiration and mentor! They both loved living The Bragg Healthy Lifestyle and inspiring millions to health.

Liquefy or Juice Fresh Organic Fruits & Vegetables

The juicer, food processor and blender are great for preparing foods, drinks, gentle (bland) diets and baby foods. Fibers of juiced fresh fruits and vegetables can be tolerated on most gentle diets. Any raw or cooked fruit or vegetable can be liquefied and added to broth, soups and non-dairy (soy, rice or coconut) milks. Fresh juices supercharge your energy level and boost your immune system to maximize the body's health power. You may fortify liquid meals or Bragg Smoothies with green vegetable powders, alfalfa, barley green, chlorella, spirulina and wheat grass for extra nutrition.

Fruit bears the closest relation to light. The sun pours a continuous flood of light into the fruits, and they furnish the best potion of food a human being requires for the sustenance of mind, body and life. – Louisa May Alcott, 1868

It's strange that some men will drink and eat anything put before them, but will check very carefully the oil they put in their car.

No man can violate Mother Nature's Laws and escape her penalties.

Fast One Day Each Week for Inner Cleansing

Fasting is the greatest cleanser and body purifier. Give it a chance to do a thorough house cleansing and help your body rid itself of accumulated toxic poisons by going on a 24- to 36-hour fast every week.

During this fast, drink 8-10 glasses of distilled water daily. Flavor with fresh lemon juice or 1-2 tsps. organic raw apple cider vinegar with 1-2 tsps. (optional) honey, maple syrup to taste or diabetics can use drop or pinch of Stevia Herb. Some add a pinch of cayenne. No food, juices or supplements are necessary.

When freed from daily chores of digesting and assimilating food, your body will use its oxygen-sparked energy to do a more thorough internal cleansing! After your first fast you will feel a renewed vitality. Make this a weekly habit and, as time goes on, you will feel even more invigorated and rejuvenated. Life is precious! Monday is our regular weekly fast day. After our evening meal on Sunday, we take in nothing but 8-10 glasses of distilled water (to 3 we add 2 tsps. of organic, raw apple cider vinegar with the 'Mother' enzyme) until Tuesday morning. We also fast the first 3 days of each month. Several times each year we do longer fasts of 7-10 days. Our favorite fast is distilled water for a week. It works wonders in keeping us fit and trim. For more information about methods and benefits of fasting, consult our book, *The Miracle of Fasting* and read the next page. (This book has changed the lives of millions worldwide. It has been a #1 seller in Russia and the Ukraine for over 40 years.)

141

Oil Pulling May Transform Your Health

The ancient Ayurvedic remedy for oral health and detoxification is oil pulling! It involves the use of pure oil – such as organic coconut oil, for pulling harmful bacteria, fungus and other organisms out of the mouth, teeth, gums and even throat. All you need to do is place about a tablespoon of oil into your mouth and swish it around for about 10-15 minutes, then please spit it out! Lipids in the oil pull out toxins and the oil absorbs toxins and bacteria. The oil helps in cellular restructuring, proper functioning of lymph nodes and other internal organs. – *OilPulling.com*

After fasting, your body becomes cleaner, stronger and full of energy.
Remember it's pollutants in the body that cause sluggishness.

BENEFITS FROM THE JOYS OF FASTING

Fasting renews your faith in yourself, your strength and God's strength.
Fasting is easier than any diet.
Fasting is the quickest way to lose weight.
Fasting is adaptable to a busy life.
Fasting gives the body a physiological rest.
Fasting is used successfully in the treatment of many physical illnesses.
Fasting can yield weight losses of up to 10 pounds or more in the first week.
Fasting lowers and normalizes cholesterol, homocysteine, blood pressure levels.
Fasting improves dietary habits.
Fasting increases pleasure eating healthy foods.
Fasting is a calming experience, often relieving tension and insomnia.
Fasting frequently induces feelings of happy euphoria, a natural high.
Fasting is a miracle rejuvenator, helps in slowing the ageing process.
Fasting is a natural stimulant to rejuvenate the growth hormone levels.
Fasting is an energizer, not a debilitator.
Fasting aids the elimination process.
Fasting often results in a more vigorous happy marital relationship.
Fasting can eliminate smoking, drug and drinking addictions.
Fasting is a regulator, educating the body to consume food only as needed.
Fasting saves precious time spent on marketing, preparing and eating.
Fasting rids the body of toxins, giving it an internal shower and cleansing.
Fasting does not deprive the body of essential nutrients.
Fasting can be used to uncover the sources of food allergies.
Fasting is used effectively in schizophrenia and other mental illness treatment.
Fasting under proper supervision can be tolerated easily up to four weeks.
Fasting does not accumulate appetite; hunger pangs disappear in 1-2 days.

Fasting is routine for most of the animal kingdom.
Fasting has been a common practice since the beginning of man's existence.
Fasting is practiced in all religions; the Bible alone has 74 references to fasting.
Fasting under proper conditions is absolutely safe.
Fasting is a blessing – "Fasting As A Way Of Life" – Allan Cott, M.D.
Fasting is not starving, it's nature's cure that God has given us. – Patricia Bragg

Dear Health Friend,

This gentle reminder explains the great benefits from "The Miracle of Fasting" that you will enjoy when starting on your weekly 24-hour Bragg Fasting Program for Super Health! It's a precious time of body-mind-soul cleansing and renewal.

On fast days I drink 8-10 glasses of distilled (our favorite) or purified water, (I add 1-2 tsps. organic apple cider vinegar to three of them). If just starting, you may also try herbal teas or try diluted fresh juices with 1/3 distilled water. Every day, even on fast days, add 1 Tbsp. of psyllium husk powder to liquids once daily. It's an extra cleanser and helps normalize weight, cholesterol and blood pressure and helps promote healthy elimination. Fasting is the oldest, most effective healing method known to man. Fasting offers great miraculous blessings from Mother Nature and our Creator. It begins the self-cleansing of the inner-body workings so we can promote our own self-healing.

My father and I wrote the book "The Miracle of Fasting" to share with you the health miracles it can perform in your life. It's all so worthwhile to do. It's an important part of The Bragg Healthy Lifestyle.

With Love,

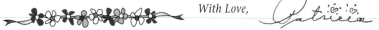

Paul Bragg's work on fasting and water is one of the great contributions to the healing wisdom and the natural health movement in the world today.
– Gabriel Cousens, M.D., author "Conscious Eating" and "Spiritual Nutrition"

Food and Product Summary

Today, sadly many foods are highly processed or refined, robbing them of essential nutrients, vitamins, minerals and enzymes. Many also contain harmful, toxic and dangerous chemicals. The research findings and experience of top nutritionists, physicians and dentists have led to the discovery that devitalized foods are a major cause of poor health, illness, cancer and premature death! The enormous increase in the last 70 years of degenerative diseases such as heart disease, arthritis, diabetes and dental decay, backs this belief. Scientific research has shown most of these afflictions can be prevented and others, once established, can be arrested or even reversed through nutritional methods – page 127.

Enjoy Super Health with Natural Foods

1. **RAW FOODS:** Fresh fruits and raw vegetables organically grown are always best! Enjoy nutritious variety garden salads with raw vegetables, sprouts, raw nuts and seeds.

2. **VEGETABLES and PROTEINS:**
   a. Legumes, lentils, brown rice, and all beans.
   b. Nuts and seeds, raw and unsalted (lightly roasted okay).
   c. We prefer healthier vegetarian proteins. If you eat animal protein, then be sure it's hormone-free, and organically fed.
   d. Dairy products – fertile range-free eggs and goat's cheese. We choose not to use dairy products. Try the healthier non-dairy: rice, coconut, oat, and almond milks.

3. **FRUITS and VEGETABLES:** Organically grown is always best – grown without the use of poisonous sprays and toxic chemical fertilizers whenever possible; do urge your markets to stock healthier organic produce! Steam, bake, sauté and stir fry vegetables as short a time as possible to retain the best nutritional content and flavor. Also enjoy fresh juices.

4. **ORGANIC non-GMO WHOLE GRAINS, CEREALS, BREADS, etc.:** Barley, rye, buckwheat, spelt, teff, oatmeal, quinoa, millet, amaranth, and wild rice contain important B-complex vitamins, vitamin E, minerals, fiber and unsaturated fatty acids.

5. **COLD or EXPELLER-PRESSED VEGETABLE OILS:** Organic, first press, extra virgin olive oil (is best), soy, flax, sunflower, and sesame oils are good sources of healthy, essential, unsaturated fatty acids. We still use oils sparingly.

HEALTHY BEVERAGES
Fresh Juices, Herb Teas & Energy Drinks

These freshly squeezed organic vegetable and fruit juices are important to *The Bragg Healthy Lifestyle*. It's not wise to drink beverages with your main meals, as it dilutes the digestive juices. But it's great during the day to have a glass of freshly squeezed orange juice, grapefruit juice, vegetable juice, raw, organic apple cider vinegar drink (see below), or herbal tea – these are all ideal pick-me-up beverages.

Apple Cider Vinegar Drink – Mix 1-2 tsps. raw, organic apple cider vinegar (with the 'Mother' enzyme) and (optional) to taste raw honey or pure maple syrup *(if diabetic, to sweeten use 2 stevia drops)* in 8 oz. of distilled or purified water. Take glass upon arising, an hour before lunch and dinner.

Delicious Hot or Cold Cider Drink – Add 2-3 cinnamon sticks and 4 cloves to water and boil. Steep 20 minutes or more. Before serving add raw organic apple cider vinegar and sweetener to taste.

Bragg's Favorite Juice Drink – This drink consists of all raw vegetables *(remember organic is best)* which we prepare in our juicer / blender: carrots, celery, cucumber, beets, cabbage, tomatoes, watercress, kale, parsley, or any vegetable combination you prefer. The great purifier, garlic we enjoy, but it's optional.

Bragg's Favorite Healthy Energy Smoothie – After our morning stretch and exercises we often enjoy the drink below instead of fruit. It's a delicious and powerfully nutritious meal anytime: lunch, dinner or in a thermos at work, school, sports, the gym and during sports or hikes. You can freeze for popsicles too.

144 Bragg's Favorite Healthy Energy Smoothie

Prepare the following in a blender, add frozen juice cubes if desired colder; Choice of: freshly squeezed orange or grapefruit juice; carrot and greens juice; unsweetened pineapple juice; or $1^1/2$ - 2 cups purified or distilled water with:

2 tsps spirulina or green powder	1-2 bananas or fresh fruit
$1/3$ tsp Nutritional Yeast	1-2 tsps almond or nut butter
2 dates or prunes-pitted	1 tsp flaxseed oil or grind seeds
1 tsp protein powder (optional)	1 tsp raw honey (optional)

Optional: 4-6 apricots (sun-dried,) soak in jar overnight in purified water or unsweetened pineapple juice. We soak enough to last for several days. Keep refrigerated. In summer you can add organic fresh fruit: peaches, papaya, blueberries, strawberries, all berries, apricots, etc. instead of banana. In winter, add apples, kiwi, oranges, tangelos, persimmons or pears, and if fresh is unavailable, try sugar-free, frozen organic fruits. Serves 1 to 2.

Patricia's Delicious Health Popcorn

Use freshly popped organic popcorn (use air popper). Drizzle organic olive oil, melted coconut oil or salt-free butter over popcorn. Sprinkle with good quality nutritional yeast for amazing flavor. For a variety try a pinch of cayenne pepper, mustard powder or fresh crushed garlic to oil mixture. Serve instead of breads!

Healthy, healing dietary fibers are organic fresh vegetables, fruits, salads whole grains and their products. These health builders help normalize your blood pressure, cholesterol and promotes healthy elimination.

Lentil & Brown Rice Casserole, Burgers or Soup
Paul Bragg and Jack LaLanne's Favorite Recipe

16 oz pkg organic lentils, uncooked
1 cup brown organic rice, uncooked
5 cups, distilled / purified water
4-6 carrots, chop $^1/_2$" rounds
3 celery stalks, chop

4 garlic cloves, chop
2 onions, chop
2 tsps organic coconut aminos
1 tsp salt-free all-purpose seasoning
2 tsps organic extra-virgin olive oil

1 cup diced fresh or canned tomatoes (salt-free)

Wash and drain lentils and rice. Place grains in large stainless steel pot. Add water, bring to boil, reduce heat and simmer 30 minutes. Now add vegetables and seasonings and cook on low heat until tender. Last five minutes add fresh or canned (salt-free) tomatoes. For delicious garnish, add minced parsley. **For Burgers mash. For Soup, add more water in cooking grains.** Serves 4 to 6.

Patricia's Raw Organic Vegetable Health Salad

2 stalks celery, chop
1 bell pepper & seeds, dice
$^1/_2$ cucumber, slice
2 carrots, grate
1 raw beet, grate
1 cup green cabbage, chop

$^1/_2$ cup red cabbage, chop
$^1/_2$ cup alfalfa, mung or sunflower sprouts
2 spring onions & green tops, chop
1 turnip, grate
1 avocado (ripe)
3 tomatoes, medium size

For variety add organic raw zucchini, peas, mushrooms, broccoli, cauliflower, (try black olives and pasta). Chop, slice or grate vegetables fine to medium for variety in size. Mix vegetables & serve on bed of lettuce, spinach, chopped kale or cabbage. Dice avocado and tomato and serve on side as a dressing. Serve choice of fresh squeezed lemon, orange or dressing separately. Chill salad plates before serving. **It's best to always eat salad first before hot dishes.** Serves 3 to 5.

145

Patricia's Health Salad Dressing

$^1/_2$ cup raw organic apple cider vinegar
1-2 tsps organic raw honey

$^1/_2$ tsp organic coconut aminos
1-2 cloves garlic, minced

$^1/_3$ cup organic extra-virgin olive oil, or blend with safflower, soy, sesame or flax oil
1 Tbsp fresh herbs, minced (to taste)

Blend ingredients in blender or jar. Refrigerate in covered jar.

For delicious Herbal Vinegar: In quart jar add $^1/_3$ cup tightly packed, crushed fresh sweet basil, tarragon, dill, oregano, or any fresh herbs desired, combined or singly (if dried herbs, use 1-2 tsps herbs). Now cover to top with raw, organic apple cider vinegar and store two weeks in warm place, and then strain and refrigerate.

Honey – Chia or Celery Seed Vinaigrette

$^1/_4$ tsp dry mustard
$^1/_4$ tsp organic coconut aminos
$^1/_4$ tsp paprika or to taste
1-2 Tbsps honey

1 cup organic apple cider vinegar
$^1/_2$ cup organic extra-virgin olive oil
$^1/_2$ small onion, minced
$^1/_3$ tsp chia or celery seed (or vary to taste)

Blend ingredients in blender or jar. Refrigerate in covered jar.

Studies show both beta carotene and vitamin C, abundantly found in fruits and vegetables, play vital roles in preventing heart disease and cancers.

MY DAILY HEALTH JOURNAL

Today is:____/____/____

> *I have said my morning resolve and am ready to practice faithfully The Bragg Healthy Lifestyle today and every day.*

Yesterday I went to bed at: Today I arose at: Weight:

Today I practiced the No-Heavy Breakfast or No-Breakfast Plan: ☐ yes ☐ no

- For Breakfast I drank: Time:

  For Breakfast I ate:
                                                            Time:

  Supplements:

- For Lunch I ate: Time:

  Supplements:

- For Dinner I ate: Time:

  Supplements:

- ____ Glasses of Water I Drank during the Day, including ACV Drinks

  List Snacks – Kind and When:

  _____
- I took part in these physical activities (walking, gym, etc.) today:

  _____

Grade each on scale of 1 to 10 (desired optimum health is 10).
- I rate my day for the following categories:

  Previous Night's Sleep: Stress/Anxiety:
  Energy Level: Elimination:
  Physical Activity, Exercise: Health:
  Peacefulness: Accomplishments:
  Happiness: Self-Esteem:
  _____

- General Comments, Reactions and any To-Do List:

Chapter 18

The Power of Vitamins

Eating healthy organic foods gives you more nutrients, super oxygen, energy and health.

Organic vegetables, fruits and grains are rich in nutrients and vitamins and contain large amounts of life-giving oxygen! Their juices are very rich in oxygen and distilled water which is Mother Nature's purest liquid!

Organic green leafy vegetables also supply organic iron, copper and other important vital minerals that are needed to manufacture hemoglobin in red blood cells. These enable the blood to absorb oxygen from the lungs and transport it to every part of your entire body.

Some cooked foods (grains, legumes, potatoes, vegetables, etc.) enhance a well-balanced healthy diet. Cooking can reduce, and in some cases, even eliminate the vitamin content. Don't overcook! We suggest you lightly steam, bake, broil or stir-fry foods that need some cooking. 147

Vitamins That Help the Respiratory System

Vitamins play a vital role in keeping our respiratory system healthy and help in reducing the risk of diseases, such as **chronic obstructive pulmonary disease (COPD), emphysema, bronchitis, pneumonia and asthma.** Chronic lower respiratory diseases are the fourth leading cause of death in the U.S. If you are considering taking vitamins that can help with respiratory problems, talk with your doctor first to determine the best course of action.

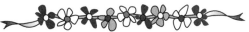

Organic, non-GMO whole grain products are excellent sources of natural vitamin E, magnesium, selenium and vital nutrients important for maintaining a healthy heart and strong bones. Shocking studies found over 80% of nutrients are lost in refining grains into white flour!

Taking natural vitamins, minerals, trace minerals and herbs are healthy added insurance to help meet the bodies daily supplemental needs.

Studies show Vitamin C and E help alleviate severity of asthma symptoms.
– Life Extension Magazine (www.lef.org)

Vitamin A – for Healthy Respiratory System

Vitamin A is a fat soluble vitamin. It has an essential role in stimulating your immune system and fighting infections. Vitamin A also assists in maintaining normal vital lung function. It repairs and strengthens mucous membranes lining the lungs. Vitamin A maintains normal functioning of mucous membrane cells that protect the lungs from harmful airborne pathogens. Individuals with lung issues that hamper breathing can benefit by increasing vitamin A intake. (See web: *LiveStrong.com*)

Vitamin A deficiencies can be damaging to the lungs, as revealed through animal testing and studies. Vitamin A deficiencies can also increase your risk of respiratory infections. Research has revealed that the lower the Vitamin A in umbilical cord blood at the time of birth, the higher the risk of lower respiratory tract infections in preschool children between one month to five years of age.

Folate and B Vitamins Boosts Immune System

148

Folate is a water soluble B vitamin that stimulates DNA production and cell reproduction. A folate deficiency can lead to an increase in the risk of respiratory diseases and infections. Researchers found that a folate deficiency in young children is an independent risk factor for lower respiratory tract infections. Scientists also discovered that children who are breastfed have a lower risk of folate deficiency and respiratory tract infections.

Our body depends on vitamin B12 to produce healthy red blood cells (RBCs). Inadequate vitamin B12 lowers RBC count, a condition called anemia, that often leads to fatigue and breathing problems, which aggravates while exercising. RBCs perform the important job of delivering oxygen to each and every cell in the body. No wonder, a vitamin B12 deficiency reduces oxygen flow to the body, resulting in shortness of breath. So, its intake may help to overcome breathing problems. Other Studies have shown that adequate levels of vitamin B6 in the blood can improve breathing, as well as significantly reduce the risk of lung cancer (*www.health.harvard.edu*).

Vitamin C Reduces Inflammation

Vitamin C is a water soluble vitamin that stimulates the immune system and protects cells from harmful substances. Increasing your dietary intake of vitamin C helps reduce the risk of respiratory infections. Studies report vitamin C supplementation can reduce the common cold by 45-91%, and helps lower the incidence of pneumonia by 80-100%.

Vitamin C can help reduce tightening of the air passages, that usually happens during or shortly after exercising. This condition referred to as exercise-induced bronchoconstriction (EIB) causes airways to become inflamed, thereby restricting free air flow into the lungs. EIB is typically marked by coughing, wheezing, and breathing trouble! Studies suggests vitamin C reduces the inflammatory response that helps alleviate EIB.

Vitamin D – Improves Exercising Performance

A supplemental dosage of vitamin D plays a crucial role in enhancing respiratory muscle function and exercise performance in COPD patients! These patients were able to exercise with more vigor and intensity due to vitamin D. Even exercising for a short duration makes these patients gasp for breath. However, increasing their vitamin D intake helps COPD patients improve their breathing and exercise performance (page 174).

Sunshine Vitamin D3 – Essential for Health

Vital vitamin D3 is a natural hormone and like other hormones it is manufactured in the body. It helps the body utilize calcium and phosphorus to build bones and teeth. Vitamin D3 also helps skin heal and boosts the immune system. Statistics from a California survey of American women found women with higher sun exposure and those with a high dietary intake of vitamin D3, had a lower risk of breast cancer. Evidence also points to a link between vitamin D3 and a reduced risk of colon cancer and bone fractures.

Skin produces approx 10,000 IUs of Vitamin D3 in response to 20-30 minutes in gentle sun exposure without using sunblock lotions.

There is evidence supporting the near-miraculous healing power of Vitamin D3, a nutrient that is available free just by enjoying gentle sunlight on your skin. Small amounts of gentle sunlight on your skin cells cause them to manufacture vitamin D3. Even as little as 10 to 20 minutes, 2 to 3 times a week should be sufficient to meet your needs. Sunscreen can reduce or even shut down the synthesis of vitamin D3, so we recommend exposure to gentle early morning or late afternoon rays without use of sunscreen! People under 50 years need 1,000 IUs, 50-70 years need 2,000 IUs and those over 70 need 2,000-5,000 IUs of vitamin D3 daily, more in special cases. Older people's abilities to produce vitamin D3 from sunlight declines. That's why it's important for those over 70 to get vitamin D3 from supplements and foods: wheat germ, raw sunflower seeds, cod liver oil, sweet potatoes, corn bread, eggs, alfalfa, saltwater fish, sardines, salmon, tuna, liver and natural vegetable oils are good sources of vitamin D3.

 Of an analysis of more that 15,000 Americans, those with low blood levels of Vitamin D3 were 30% more likely to have high blood pressure, 40% more apt to have high triglycerides, 98% more likely to be diabetic and 129% more apt to be obese! Researchers noted that low Vitamin D3 may also be a culprit for Fibromyalgia, Multiple Sclerosis, Rheumatoid Arthritis and other joint diseases.

Five Ways Vitamin D3 Can Save Your Life

1. **Promotes Weight Loss:** You need Vitamin D3 to effectively help you lose weight. Your insulin works better and Vitamin D3 helps you lose belly fat. Diabetes is also related to low Vitamin D3 levels.

2. **Reduces Risk of Early, Pre-mature Death.**

3. **Fewer Bone Fractures**: Without Vitamin D3, calcium can't be absorbed. But if you get enough vitamin D3, it can help you avoid osteoporosis, bone fractures and falling, which are causes of death among the elderly.

4. **Reduces Risk of Heart Disease:** Vitamin D3 improves blood flow by relaxing blood vessels and lowering blood pressure.

5. **Helps Fight Cancer:** D3 improves the functioning of your immune system and that helps fight cancer!

Five Ways To Get Vitamin D3

1. **15 minutes of high-noon sun exposure** in warmer climates a few times a week. *(We prefer early or late sun.)*

2. **Fatty Fish and Cod Liver Oil:** If you have been warned to stay out of the sun, another good source of Vitamin D3 is oily fish, such as salmon, tuna, mackerel and trout.

3. **Enjoy mushrooms, orange juice and almond milk.**

4. **Multi-Vitamin Supplements**: Most all multi-vitamins have a substantial amount of vitamin D3.

5. **Vitamin D Supplements:** 1000 to 2000 IUs Vitamin D3 recommended daily *(seniors 2000 - 3000 IUs, page 150).*

Vitamin E – A Powerful Antioxidant

Vitamin E provides significant protective effects against a wide range of respiratory disorders, including COPD. Taking vitamin E can help repair lung tissue and even rebuild lung capacity, in turn easing breathing problems. Vitamin E also protects the lungs by nullifying the impact of inhaled pollutants. The possibility of using vitamin E as an *antidote to smog* has been well researched. Dr. Al (Aloys) L. Tappel, Biochemistry Professor, University of California, Davis, stated that the natural antioxidation property of vitamin E helps reverse the ageing process. He recommended vitamin E supplements for everyone to help promote a healthier, longer life. *For more suggestions on natural supplements and herbs read pages 31 and 36.*

151

Add Wonder-Working Vitamin E Tocotrienols

E Tocotrienols provide greater antioxidant protection against lipid peroxidation than standard vitamin E. This oxygen conserving ability of vitamin E Tocotrienols may be effective in relief of emphysema, the deadly disease of lung deterioration which has increased as our air has become more contaminated. Another vitamin E healing gift is its oil as an amazingly effective skin treatment for home application to minor burns, sunburn, skin rashes, scars, and even stretch marks.

Miracle natural vitamin E Tocotrienols supplements are available at health stores. If just starting vitamin E, doctors recommend you begin with 100 IUs daily. Gradually increase to 800 IUs for women and 1200 IUs for men.

Organic Non-GMO Whole Grains Sustain Life

When you buy bread, be sure to select only 100% organic non-GMO whole grain breads. It's fun to bake your own. We try to bake a delicious variety of breads once a week.

Another good food source of vitamin E and nutrients is cornmeal mush (below) made with organic stoneground yellow cornmeal from health stores (not the refined, degerminated variety found in commercial stores).

Bragg Family's Favorite Cornmeal Recipe

*1 cup organic cornmeal yellow stoneground
3 to 3 1/2 cups distilled water
3 Tbsps raisins, sliced prunes or dates (optional)
1 Tbsp Organic Nut Butter* for topping (optional)*

152

Moisten meal with 2 cups cold water. Boil balance of water, then slowly add moistened cornmeal and raisins. Mix well. When evenly thickened, place in top of double boiler (or put pot in pan of water) with low heat so not to burn! Cook 15 minutes. Serve hot. Top with honey, blackstrap molasses, agave nectar or 100% pure maple syrup (our favorite) and sliced fresh organic fruit (banana, apples, berries, peaches are delicious). Optional toppings: rice, almond or coconut milks, even nut butter.

Note: If you are serving this to only a few people, there might be some left over. Put in a flat pan, cool and refrigerate. For breakfast or a main meal, slice and dip in egg (use fertile, free range) batter, and roll in wheat germ flakes. Lightly sauté in olive oil. Serve hot. For variety this cornmeal is delicious topped with a poached egg and a little 100% pure maple syrup.

*Organic Nut Butters (almond, peanut, etc.) are delicious in oatmeal and hot cereals, stir in cereal just before serving. (For delicious homemade organic nut butters see page 124.)

Vitamin E protects cells from damaging free radical effects which damage cells and might contribute to development of heart disease and cancer.
– ods.od.nih.gov

Vitamin E-Rich Healthy Foods Are Important For Your Health

Here's a list of healthy foods that contain the following notable amounts of precious Vitamin E. Buy organic sources – they are best! Reference from The National Institutes of Health.

Food	Quantity	Vitamin E IU's
Apples	1 medium	1.21
Almonds	1/4 cup	13.37
Bananas	1 medium	0.40
Barley	1/2 cup	4.20
Beans, navy	1/2 cup	3.60
Bell Peppers	1 cup slices	0.94
Blueberries	1 cup	2.18
Broccoli	1 cup	1.12
Butter (salt-free)	6 tablespoons	2.40
Carrots	1 cup	0.45
Celery, green	1/2 cup	2.60
Corn oil	1 tablespoon	2.83
Eggs, fertile	2	2.62
Grapefruit	1/2	0.52
Kale	1/2 cup	8.00
Lettuce	6 leaves	0.50
Olive Oil (virgin)	1 tablespoon	2.38
Onions, raw	2 medium	0.26
Oranges	1 small	0.24
Papaya	1 medium	5.06
Peas, green	1 cup	4.00
Potatoes, white	1 medium	0.06
Potatoes, sweet	1 small	4.00
Rice, brown	1 cup cooked	2.40
Rye	1/2 cup	3.00
Soybean Oil	1 tablespoon	2.24
Sunflower Seeds, raw	1 oz.	8.94
Tomato	1 medium	1.01
Wheat Germ Oil	1 tablespoon	26.20

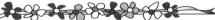

From a revealing study of nurses whose daily intake of Vitamin E was 800 IU's and more, 36% had an amazingly lower risk of dangerous heart attacks and 23% had a lower risk of strokes!

Locations in the Body Where Osteoporosis, Arthritis, Pain and Misery Hit the Hardest

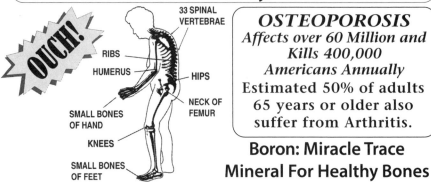

OSTEOPOROSIS
Affects over 60 Million and Kills 400,000 Americans Annually
Estimated 50% of adults 65 years or older also suffer from Arthritis.

Boron: Miracle Trace Mineral For Healthy Bones

BORON – An important trace mineral for healthier and stronger bones that also helps the body absorb more vital calcium, minerals and necessary hormones! Good Boron sources are most organic veggies, fresh and sun-dried fruits, avocados, prunes, raw nuts and soybeans.

The U.S. Dept. of Agriculture's Nutrition Lab in Grand Forks, ND, says Boron is usually found in soil and foods, but many Americans eat a diet low in Boron. They conducted a 17 week study which showed a daily 3 to 6 mgs. Boron supplement enabled participants to reduce loss (demineralization) of calcium, phosphorus and magnesium from their bodies. This loss is usually caused by eating processed fast foods, drinking tap waters (distilled is best), eating lots of meat, salt, sugar and fat and a dietary lack of fresh vegetables, fruits and whole grains. (*all-natural.com*)

Scientific studies show women benefit from a healthy lifestyle that includes vitamin D3 sunshine and exercise (even weight-lifting) to maintain healthier bones, combined with distilled water, low-fat, high-fiber, carbohydrate, and fresh organic fruits, salads, sprouts, greens and vegetable diet. This lifestyle helps protect against heart disease, high blood pressure, cancer and many other ailments! I'm happy to see science now agrees with my father who first stated these health truths in 1920's.

For more hormone and osteoporosis facts, read pioneer, Dr. John Lee's book – "What Your Doctor May Not Tell You About Menopause"

Boron helps keep skeletal structure strong by adding to bone density, preventing Osteoporosis, treating Arthritis and improving strength and muscle mass. Boron helps facilitate calcium directly into the bones. Boron protects bones by regulating Estrogen function. Boron is naturally found in beans, nuts, avocados, berries, plums, oranges and grapes. Boron helps relieve menopause symptoms and PMS. – Dr. Axe

Chapter 19

Doctor Rest – The Recharger of Life

Doctor Rest is another health specialist always at your command to help you achieve Supreme Vitality and Health! We believe the word *rest* is the most misunderstood word in the English language. Some people's idea of resting is to sit down and drink a cup of a strong stimulant such as coffee, black tea or caffeinated soft drinks. This is typified by the *coffee break*. To us, rest means repose, freedom from activity and quiet tranquility. It means peace of mind and spirit. It means to rest without anxiety or worry! Rest means to refresh and should renew your whole nervous system and your entire body – physically, mentally, and spiritually.

When you're resting, you shouldn't sit with one leg crossed over the other because this position puts a heavy burden on the popliteal artery which supplies the feet with blood and also cuts off nerve energy. If you sit with legs crossed you are not resting, but giving your heart an extra load of work to do! When you sit down, it's best to keep both feet on the floor or a footstool (see page 167).

To rest means to allow free circulation (no restrictions) of blood throughout the body, which is important for health. Are your shoes too tight? Your collar? Your hat? Your stockings? Your watch, belt, undergarments, bra*****? If yes, then you're not resting when you sit or lie down!

Why do we rest? Often people say, *"I need to rest!"* Yet when they sit down intending to rest, they nervously drum their fingers on a table or desk, quiver or shake their legs or squirm and move about restlessly.

The art of resting is something that must be acquired and concentrated upon! The best rest can only be secured when your body is relaxed and freed from restrictive clothing! Your clothes should be comfortably loose.

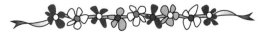

*Read "Dressed To Kill" by S. Singer, on breast cancer and bra studies.
Women, please cut wires out of bras that hinder your circulation!
I prefer not to wear a bra but instead a loose chemise. – Patricia Bragg

Enjoy Rest & Naps – It's Not a Crime to Relax!

One good way to rest is to lie down on a firm bed, unclothed or wearing as few, loose clothes as possible. Another way to rest is to sunbathe, see pages 187-190. There is nothing that will relax the muscles and nerves like the gentle, soothing early morning or late afternoon sunrays. In order to rest and nap, you must learn to clear your mind of all anxiety, worries and emotional problems. When the muscles and nerves are relaxed, the heart action slows – especially when you take long, slow, deep breaths! This will help promote a deeper relaxation and increased rest that promotes more total health!

Another good form of resting is a short nap. When you take a nap, command your muscles to become completely relaxed. Your conscious and subconscious mind control the muscles and the nerves, so you must be in complete command of your body when you rest.

Sleep – The Body's Miracle Recharger

Sleep is the greatest revitalizer we have, but few people get a long, peaceful, refreshing night's sleep. Most people habitually use stimulants: tobacco, drugs, coffee, tea and other caffeinated drinks, which batter tired nerves! People who use these toxic stimulants never have complete rest and relaxation because nerves are always in an excited condition.

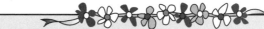

Say Good-bye to Tiredness – Hello Super Energy

- Sit down and kick off your shoes. Let tiredness go away and relax!
- Now start breathing in easily and deeply, then breathe out tiredness. Next breathe deeply in a feeling of complete peace and relaxation.
- Curl your toes down tight, now relax toes and feet. Repeat exercise: Now tighten, then relax fingers and slowly do arms, legs, butt, etc.
- Breathe out slowly all the pressures and tiredness of the day. Then breathe in refreshing joy, health, love and peace.
- Now relax, close eyes for 10 minutes, then after stand up and stretch.
- Stand, stretch arms up, now do wide windmill circles, then reverse circles.
- Now stretch your body, arms and legs – sideways, up and down, etc.

Breathe deeply in new life – breathe out stress and tension

Most people do not earn their rest. Rest must be earned with physical and mental activity, because they go hand in hand. So many people complain what poor sleepers they are – that they toss and turn throughout the night. For an extra relaxer before bedtime try an apple cider vinegar drink, hot or cold, it's delicious; see recipe on page 144. (More on sleep pages 91-100.)

Sadly millions take some type of drug or alcohol to induce sleep, but this is not true sleep! No one gets restful sleep with sleeping drugs or alcohol. You may drug yourself into unconsciousness, but that very drug will deprive you of a normal, restful, recharging sleep.

Healthy Lifestyle Promotes Sound Sleep

Your nerves are continually irritated when you do not eliminate the toxins from your body. How is it possible to get a good night's rest with irritated nerves? When we faithfully live our Bragg Healthy Lifestyle, exercise, breathe deeply and perform weekly 24-hour fasts, we enjoy and earn sound sleep! We discovered that when our students discard their stimulants and begin a regular fasting program, they too enjoy a more restful, deep sleep. **157**

You will notice as you purify your body that you will be able to relax more readily. You will be able to enjoy naps and you will reap the benefits of a long, restful, night's sleep. Rest is important!

Life is to be Savored and Enjoyed – Not Hectic

Today we live in a hectic, competitive environment, which the business world calls the *rat race*. During these stressful times filled with political and emotional unrest, we build up tremendous pressures, tensions and strains. This is why people turn to tobacco, drugs, coffee, alcohol and other harmful substances – to try to escape the stress.

Follow Mother Nature and God – rewards are great! – Patricia Bragg

Lavender helps you relax. Before drying off after your nightly bath or shower, place three drops of lavender essential oil on a damp washcloth and rub it gently over your body. The soothing active agents in the lavender oil will enter into your body through your skin and nose.

There is not only competition in the business world, but in family and social realms as well, as people strive to maintain their *status*. People are always trying to impress one another and trying to create a certain *image*. Often they create a false image and it takes energy to portray this falseness! There is tremendous pressure on people who believe their worth is being dependent on their appearance. So they spend hours primping and posing constantly trying to keep up with the latest fads, struggling to have a different – *perfect* – body. All of this calls for energy. Our modern civilization drives and pushes us, robbing us of our natural, peaceful state.

It's no wonder we have created millions of alcoholics and drug addicts! Why have people completely forgotten that life is meant to be lived and enjoyed? Too few individuals these days enjoy leisure living. Life is one big rush! Where and why is everyone rushing these days? It's best to slow down, relax – get healthy and be happy!!!

To be able to relax, rest and sleep you must schedule your day so you have balanced time for work, rest, recreation, exercise and then a good night's sleep. Also, you can't get a good sleep if you overload your stomach! You will enjoy better sleep if you earn it with daily exercise, brisk walking, gardening, etc. We have fondness and concern for you and love being your health teachers and friends to inspire you to live The Bragg Healthy Lifestyle! Please nourish your body with healthy natural foods, pure distilled water, lots of fresh air, exercise and deep breathing exercises.

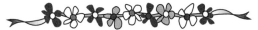

I have the wisdom of my years and youthfulness of The Bragg Healthy Lifestyle. I never act or feel my calendar years! I feel ageless! So why shouldn't you? Start living this Bragg Healthy Way today! – Patricia Bragg

Start being happier, smile and laugh more, it's up to you! Healthy actions speak louder than words and can elevate your mood if you feel depressed. Take a brisk walk in a natural setting and practice slow, deep breathing – it helps you sort out and solve problems. Find something funny to read and laugh about. As often as possible make yourself smile and laugh; it opens blood vessels in the back of your head to physically lift your mood. No one "makes" you happy – it's an inner attitude that sparkles from within.

Love Mother Nature and Yourself Daily

Enjoy a balanced program of exercise and repose and let Mother Nature do the rest! Treat yourself as you deserve to be treated and the results will astound you! We, the *Back to Nature People*, have been ridiculed for years as faddists and extremists. Now our healthy lifestyle is in demand! The popular press prints stories daily confirming what we have always known! We believe in Mother Nature and want to spread her health, joy, peace, happiness and love worldwide.

We recommend that you return to a more natural way of living in food, clothing, rest and in simplicity of lifestyle habits. Strive for harmony with Mother Nature. Live as Mother Nature wants. Realize that she loves you and you are part of her family. Put yourself in her hands and let her inner wisdom guide you. Mother Nature is eager to inspire and guide you so she can help you perfect your human machine. She can help cleanse, heal and improve your body if you work with her by living a healthier life! Please follow The Bragg Healthy Lifestyle.

Aromatherapy – A Healer For Centuries

Aromatherapy is the practice of using natural oils extracted from flowers, leaves, bark or other parts of a plant to enhance psychological and physical well-being. The inhaled aroma from these "essential" oils is widely believed to stimulate brain function. Essential oils can also be absorbed through the skin, where they travel through the bloodstream and can promote whole-body healing. Aromatherapy has the power to work miracles, to uplift and heal. Treat yourself to the delights and fragrances of essential oils. Smelling beautiful roses, flowers and fruit blossoms is also recharging.
See more info on Aromatherapy on page 194. – (*AromaTherapy.com*)

HAVE AN ATTITUDE OF GRATITUDE: Gratitude creates happiness because it makes us feel full and complete. Gratitude is the realization that we have everything we need! One of the truths about gratitude is that it's impossible to feel both the positive emotion of thankfulness and a negative emotion such as anger or fear at the same time. Gratitude gives only positive feelings – love, compassion, joy and hope. As we focus on what we are thankful for fear, anger and unhappy thoughts simply melt away.
– Excerpt from "Attitudes of Gratitude" by M.J. Ryan

When possible, leave the smog-filled, air-polluted cities for the country. In the quiet beauty of meadows and hills, you will rekindle your youth. For success: plan, plot and follow through with a strong belief you will become healthier and more youthful! If you live in a city, make it a point to go enjoy your parks, the country, walk the hills, valleys, or the seashore where you can find clean air and relaxation, in a peaceful natural setting for beautiful, recharging retreat time for your body, mind and soul.

Wise Tips for Healthy, Peaceful Living

• Regard your body as a wonderful miracle machine, 100% under your care and control! Become your own health captain and guardian of your habits of living so you may be well balanced for a long lifetime of health.

• Demand of yourself a higher standard of healthy lifestyle habits! Recognize that every machine must have rest periods! You can't receive higher, super health unless your body gets its rest periods to develop new found vitality and boundless energy! Without sufficient rest, health problems build up when your vital nerve force is depleted. Sadly a majority of Americans are stressed-out and unhealthy. Read our *Building Powerful Nerve Force & Positive Energy* book (see back pages for book list) for more info about building powerful, healthy, peaceful nerves.

• You will become wiser and more mature when you draw closer to and become more intimate with God and Mother Nature! Stop seeking over-stimulation and thrills; instead, seek a simple, "back to nature" peaceful life! Be faithful and you will have a healthy, long and active life as Mother Nature intended for you to enjoy.

Man's days shall be 120 years. – Genesis 6:3

You are encircled by the arms of the mystery of God. – Hildegard of Bingen

Just by paying attention to breathing, you can access new levels of health and relaxation that will benefit every area of your life. – Deepak Chopra, M.D.

Romance with Mother Nature never grows stale, she walks with you and talks with you and her wisdom is thrilling! – Patricia Bragg

Dream big, think big and enjoy the many miracles.

Chapter 20

The Importance of Doctor Good Posture

Sit, stand and walk tall for super health!

Humans – from head to feet – are built to stand, sit and walk erect. Now that we have reviewed the way your breathing apparatus operates, you can readily understand how correct posture is essential to correct breathing. When you slump, you squeeze your vital organs and lungs into a cramped position that seriously limits the operation of your diaphragm. You become a shallow breather, able to use only the top portion of your lungs. When you sit bent over a desk, you rob your body of maximal oxygen intake, impair circulation, hamper the functions of your heart and vital organs and crowd your muscles and bones into unnatural positions! Then you wonder why you're so fatigued! You probably also cross your legs, which further blocks circulation, preparing the way for broken capillaries, varicose veins, backaches, **161** headaches and a host of unhealthy problems.

It is likely that you maintain the same poor posture when on your feet – standing or walking with your shoulders and head drooping forward. You cannot improve matters by suddenly going to the opposite extreme: distorting your body and all of its components by an exaggerated reversal (i.e., thrusting shoulders back and sucking in stomach). You can and will improve and maintain good posture by strengthening your muscles with daily exercise and by practicing correct posture habits daily! *Start now – it works miracles!*

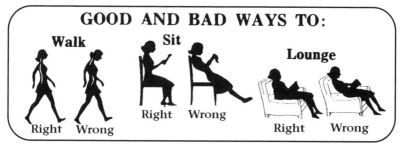

GOOD AND BAD WAYS TO:

Walk   **Sit**   **Lounge**

Right   Wrong   Right   Wrong   Right   Wrong

Poor posture can decrease breathing capacity by as much as 30%!
That means there's 30% less oxygen getting to your brain and other cells.

Posture Can Make or Break Your Health!

Why should emphasis be placed upon such a simple thing as the pull of gravity? In your youth, your muscles held your skeleton in proper balance free from strain or discomfort. Perhaps now circumstances have caused your muscles to lose the battle with gravity. Maybe premature ageing, excess weight or an enforced rest has weakened your muscles just enough to cause your frame to be in an uncomfortable state of balance.

PERFECT POSTURE AND ALIGNMENT

This sagging stretches the ligaments of your back and causes backaches, and when stretched too far they become painful. They are meant to serve only as a check point for the joints and cannot be forcibly stretched without pain. When the ligaments in your back are made uncomfortable by excessive stretching, it is natural for your muscles to try to oppose this gravitational pull. However, if your muscles are too weak to do their proper job, they will rapidly become exhausted and develop the misery of fatigue, making your back painful and uncomfortable.

162

Check your own symptoms! Do you notice a deep aching and soreness along your spine due to stretched ligaments? Are your back and shoulder muscles achy and tired? Do you have a postural backache caused by weak muscles and bad posture? If so, start now to strengthen your muscles with proper posture and exercise.

Your Health Friend is Doctor Posture

Look at yourself in the mirror! Do your shoulders slump? Is your upper back round? Do you have a potbelly? Are you swaybacked? Can you see the reasons why your back has the right to ache? The bending, slumping, ligament-stretching force of gravity has finally taken charge. Even though you might be a sufferer of backaches due to poor muscles and bad posture, don't despair. With good exercise

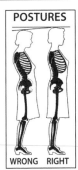

POSTURES

WRONG   RIGHT

and good posture habits, plus living The Bragg Healthy Lifestyle you can regain your back and joint comfort!

WHERE DO YOU STAND?

POSTURE CHART

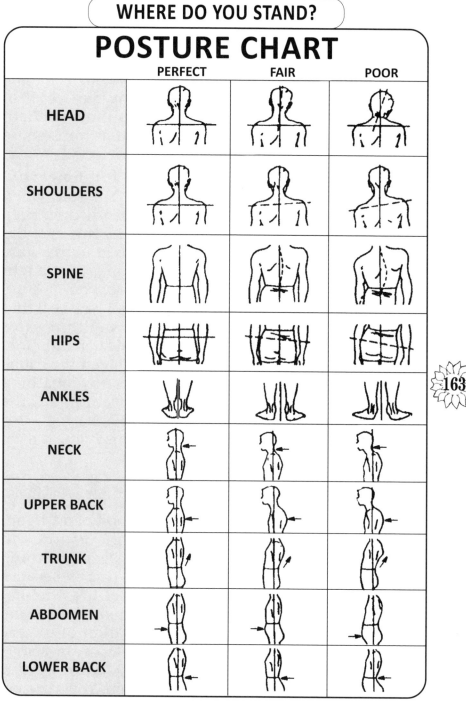

	PERFECT	FAIR	POOR
HEAD			
SHOULDERS			
SPINE			
HIPS			
ANKLES			
NECK			
UPPER BACK			
TRUNK			
ABDOMEN			
LOWER BACK			

163

Your posture carries you through life from your head to your feet. This is your human vehicle and you are truly a miracle! Cherish, respect and protect it by living The Bragg Healthy Lifestyle. – Patricia Bragg

Remember – Your posture can make or break your looks and health!

Good Posture – First Step to Healthy Living

Poor posture puts your heart, lungs and all of your *working machinery* into a viselike grip which impairs operations, circulation and efficiency. Keep saying to yourself, *"I must stretch up tall and lift up my chest and diaphragm."* Now, you will be exercising during all of your waking hours. Good posture brings inner strength and tone to your organs and muscles that no exercise can provide.

Correct posture is vital for health and longevity! Keep a straight line from the chin to the toes when standing. Don't slump in your chair when sitting. Keep the head, chest and diaphragm held high. This may tire you at first, but only because your unused muscles are being re-awakened and trained! Once you give strength and tone to the many muscles that control your posture (some also help hold your internal organs), you will find it's easy to maintain good posture. The health rewards are many and you will look and feel healthier and more youthful. Relearning correct posture and breathing habits helps you to attain and maintain the healthy breathing practices you had as a baby. You must learn to breathe with every cell of your lungs. It is then that you can raise your rate of physical vibration to its highest level for super energy and vitality.

Normalize Figure with Good Posture & Exercise

You can actually create a more fit body and figure by using correct posture and breathing exercises and living The Bragg Healthy Lifestyle. All deep breathing exercises are body-building exercises. This is because oxygen is the invisible food – the staff of life, the life-giving miracle force of the body's 75 trillion cells and the vital compliment of the body's assimilation of dietary food. These exercises will help build up a person who is underweight and trim down a person who is overweight. You can burn off fat by internal combustion. You can tone your body and keep it that way. Start now to normalize your figure into its naturally pleasing curves with correct deep breathing habits, along with brisk walking, regular exercise and healthy, wholesome food.

Bragg Posture Exercise Brings Miracles
Do This Exercise Daily and Practice Good Posture!

Stand tall with feet 9-12" apart. Tighten your butt and suck in stomach muscles. Lift up rib cage, stretch up spine, hold chest up, shoulders back and lift chin up slightly. Line up your spine – put finger on nose, plumb line straight to belly button, drop arms to sides and swing them to normalize your posture. Look in the mirror to see improvements. Do this posture exercise often; wonderful changes will occur! You are retraining and strengthening your muscles to stand straight for a healthier, fit body with more energy and youthfulness. Stand, walk and sit tall!

Wear Loose, Comfortable Clothing

Don't spoil your health with restrictive clothing such as tight belts, collars, undergarments, bras (page 155) and even tight shoes for they can hamper breathing, blood circulation and the functioning of major organs. It can also throw your body and posture off balance.

Which Posture Do You Have?

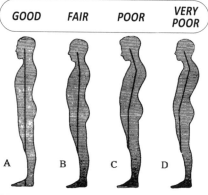

GOOD   FAIR   POOR   VERY POOR

A   B   C   D

A) GOOD: Head, trunk, thigh in straight line; chest high and forward; abdomen flat; and back curves normal.

B) FAIR: Head forward; abdomen prominent; exaggerated curve in upper back; slightly hollowed back.

C) POOR: Relaxed (fatigued) posture; head forward and down; abdomen relaxed; shoulder blades prominent; hollowed back.

D) VERY POOR: Head forward and down; exaggerated curve in upper back; abdomen relaxed; chest flat-sloping; hollowed back.

How we stand and how we sit affects how we breathe. If the body is slumped over, the shoulders become rounded and the rib cage collapses, giving the lungs no room to expand. Notice the difference in your ability to breathe deeply when you are slumped over a desk or when you are sitting erectly, giving the lungs a chance for maximum expansion.

He who breathes the most air, lives the better life. – Elizabeth Barrett Browning

Learn to Stand, Sit and Walk Tall
For Body Strength and Super Health

To maintain and keep in a healthy state involves many factors including healthy natural food, deep breathing, exercise, rest, sleep, control of emotions and mind, fasting and good posture. If you nourish and give your body loving care, good posture is natural. Conversely, when your body lacks any of these essentials, poor posture is usually the result. Once you have established poor habits, you will have to take definite and corrective measures! You will need to exercise regularly and practice good postural habits in order to restore your natural, healthy stature.

When you sit, your spine should be straight against the chair and both feet should be squarely on floor or foot stool. Your abdominal cavity should be drawn in. Keep shoulders back and hold your chest and head high, never forward. Your arms may be relaxed or lightly clasped in your lap.

When you walk, imagine that your legs are attached to the middle of your chest. This will give you long, gliding, graceful steps. When you walk correctly with this swing and spring, you will naturally build energy. **Your habits either make or break you! Good posture habits help make graceful, strong bodies. Remember this –**

As the twig is bent, so is the tree inclined.

When you sit, keep your torso up and relaxed. Sit squarely on your bottom (it's padded). Keep your feet flat on the floor or with ankles lightly crossed. You can work for hours at your desk in this position without fatigue, but it's best to stop hourly for a good body stretch. Stand, stretch your spine up and do some shoulder rolls forward, then backwards. Then for more energy do some arm-wide swinging windmills (see page 186). Also take frequent brisk walks, maintaining healthy posture with your arms swinging and breathing deeply in rhythm with your stride.

Poor posture can bring unbearable pain across your upper back and fatigue in your drooping shoulders. It can cause weakness in your hips and loins, a numb feeling at your tail bone and often, shooting pain down your legs. Bad posture can develop aches and pains all over the body.

Don't Cross Your Legs – It's Unhealthy

When sitting never cross your legs! Under the knees run two of the largest arteries, called popliteal arteries carrying nourishing blood to the muscles below the knees and to nerves in the feet. You immediately cut down the blood flow to a trickle when you cross your legs.

When the muscles of the legs and knees are not nourished and don't have good circulation, then the extremities stagnate, which can lead to varicose veins. Look at the ankles of people age 40 and over who have the habit of crossing their legs. Note the broken veins and capillaries. When the muscles and feet do not get their full supply of blood, the feet become weak and poor circulation sets in. Cold feet usually torment the leg-crosser.

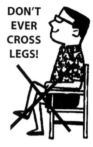

DON'T EVER CROSS LEGS!

A well-known heart specialist was asked, "When do most people have a heart attack?" He answered, "At a time they are sitting quietly with one leg crossed over the other." When you sit, plant both feet squarely on the floor or a box if needed. Crossing your legs puts an unnecessary burden on your heart!

167

People who are habitual leg-crossers have more acid crystals stored in the feet than those who never cross their legs. Crossing the legs is one of the worst postural habits of man. It throws the hips, spine and head off balance and it's the most common cause of chronic backaches, headaches and varicose veins. Be kind to your body – please don't cross your legs. You can break this bad habit.

The Dangers of Sitting Too Long

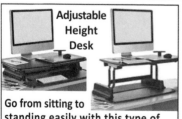

Adjustable Height Desk

Go from sitting to standing easily with this type of stand-up desk.

People who sit too long at work may develop a thrombosis (blood clot) in the deep veins of the calf. If your office work requires you to sit a lot at a computer, *get up and move around every hour ◀ or get this desk.*

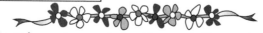

A strong body makes a strong mind. – Thomas Jefferson, 3rd U.S. President

Stand and Walk Whenever Possible!

Long amounts of sitting are bad for your health. Sitting over six hours total per day is shown to put a person at higher risk of dying from cardiovascular disease. Extended sitting slows metabolism of glucose and lowers the levels of good (HDL) cholesterol in the blood – risk factors toward developing heart disease and Type 2 Diabetes. Studies show reducing time spent sitting by only 66 minutes daily, a sedentary person can experience 54% reduction in back and neck pain and can increase life expectancy by an additional 2 years!

Over 31 Million Americans Suffer Backaches

It has been said that a backache is the penalty people must pay for the privilege of standing and walking upright on two feet. The spines of humans have normal curves that enable muscles to oppose gravity and hold the back erect. As long as the muscles are strong enough to maintain balance and prevent a sagging camel-back, the back is comfortable. When muscles are too weak to work, the back sags, ligaments are stretched and then the inevitable happens – a backache, that sadly affects millions of Americans!

Good posture is an important part of breathing. For correct posture, align your body with an imaginary vertical line from the top center of your head through the center of your pelvis to the floor between your feet. Do the Bragg Posture Exercises often, see page 60 and 165.

Now establish this simple, incredibly beneficial habit: stand tall, walk tall and sit tall. When this healthy posture becomes a habit, the result is correct posture! Any sagging, prolapsed vital organs will slowly assume and take their normal positions and function better. Daily faithfully follow The Bragg Healthy Lifestyle and drink 8 glasses of pure distilled water and always practice good posture.

Poor posture inhibits the flow of oxygen throughout the body. With less oxygen taken in, every cell in the body then becomes undernourished and hungry for fresh oxygen. Of paramount importance is the circulation to the head area. Because of gravity, blood carrying oxygen naturally has to work harder to get up above the heart into the head. When poor posture interferes with circulation it also affects skin, eyes, organs, brain, hair.
– Philip Smith, "Total Breathing"

168

Chapter 21

Doctor Fresh Air

Dr. Fresh Air is a Super Health Specialist and offers the following prescription for a long, healthy, fulfilled life:

> ### The Breath of Pure Fresh Air,
> ### Is The Invisible Staff of Life.

The first thing we do when we are born is to take a long, deep breath and the final thing we do is take a last gasp before we stop breathing and pass. Between birth and death our whole life is completely maintained by our breathing!

Dr. Fresh Air wants you to have a long, healthy life. Practice the Super Power Breathing Exercises and remain conscious that with every breath you take you are bringing precious life-giving oxygen into your body! People who fail to obey the doctor's orders about getting plenty of fresh air day and night invite many severe complications. Let us examine the function of breathing. Air is invisible food – the only food that we absolutely cannot live without! If we are deprived of air for over 5 to 7 minutes, death takes us! **We are miracle breathing machines! Nurture, protect and honor your precious life!**

Air supplies us with life-giving oxygen CO_2, which is critical for every cell in our bodies. Oxygen is carried by the blood to the lungs where miracles take place: the exchange of life-giving oxygen for deadly carbon dioxide. We create deadly toxins in the process of living that CO_2 carries out of our bodies. These are collected by our blood, brought to our lungs and expelled as the new life-giving oxygen enters our bloodstream! During the process of metabolism, the building up and tearing down of the cells of the body, and in the very process of living, carbon dioxide poison is constantly burned up and expelled.

You are what you breathe, eat, drink, think, say & do!
– Patricia Bragg, Pioneer Health Crusader

Our breathing is a miracle process to support the ongoing miracle awareness of life in running our daily lives. – Jon Kabat-Zinn, Ph.D.

169

We are Miracle Air Breathing Machines

When a person does not get enough fresh air – or is a shallow breather – and their intake of oxygen does not equal the output of carbon dioxide, this poison can then build up in the body. This could result in serious physical problems because the retained carbon dioxide can be concentrated in other parts of the body.

Enervation is the lack of nerve energy that lowers the Vital Force so much that the lungs cannot pump in enough air to flush carbon dioxide out of the body. Now you see how important it is to breathe fresh air deeply and be faithful with Super Power Breathing exercises every day!

We are air-pressure machines and oxygen purifies our bodies. It's one of the greatest detoxifiers of the human body. We live at the bottom of an atmospheric ocean approximately 70 miles deep. This air pressure is 14 lbs/sq. inch. Between the inhalation and the exhalation of a breath, a vacuum is formed. As long as we continue to have this rhythmical intake of oxygen and outflow of carbon dioxide, we will live. We know that we can go without food for 30 days or more and still survive, but we can only go without air for a few minutes. Air is one of the most important energizers of the human body. **The more deeply you breathe, the better your chances for extending your years for a long healthy life on Earth.**

For over 70 years, my father researched long-lived people and found one common factor among them: they are deep breathers! The deeper – and therefore fewer – breaths a person takes in one minute, the longer that person lives. Rapid breathers are short-lived. This holds true in the animal world, too. Rabbits, guinea pigs and all kinds of rodents are rapid breathers, taking many breaths every minute. They are among the shortest-lived creatures on the face of Earth. For years we have made it a practice to take long, slow, deep breaths when we first get up in the morning. During the day, we also try to take 3-5 minute breaks where we breathe long, deeper full breaths. Try this now – it makes you feel wonderfully alive!

Change your lifestyle to healthy living, then you will improve your life!

Indian Holy Men & Women Practice Slow, Deep Breathing and Prayer Meditation

On my father's expeditions into India, he found holy men in secluded retreats who devoted their lives to building physically powerful bodies as instruments for high spiritual advancement. They spent many hours daily in the practice of rhythmic, relaxed, long, slow, deep breathing. These holy men of India were utterly fantastic physically. The deep breathing of fresh air kept their skin and muscle-tone ageless. Dad met a holy man in the foothills of the Himalaya Mountains who told him that he was 126 years old. This man's whole life was spent getting closer to God, and he is the one who taught my father the system which we expanded upon and teach around the world . . . *The Bragg Super Power Breathing.*

This holy man had perfect vision and he had a beautiful head of hair. He had all his teeth and the endurance and stamina of an athlete. He also spoke five languages fluently. He was one of the most amazing men my father had ever met! When asked to what he owed his great strength, youthfulness and mentality, he answered, *"I have made a lifelong practice of faithfully doing my slow, deep breathing and prayer meditations daily."*

My father does not like to guess the age of any person, but while he was on this trip to India he met a woman whose age he guessed to be about 50. He was amazed when she told him she was 86. She was a beautiful woman with vitality and no sign of age deterioration! He was impressed and asked her the secret of her natural beauty and her agelessness! Again he got the same answer he did from the holy man, this beautiful woman was conscious of the importance of deep, slow breathing and prayer!

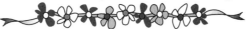

"I am not perfect. My mind wanders during my mediation practice and I sometimes feel the difficulties of life get under my skin. I know I need improvement. Happiness and well-being is a process. We make a choice about whether to try to be happy or not. Choosing happiness means cultivating your compassion, your generosity, your concern for others and continuously trying to push any negative thoughts out! The act of cultivating happiness, in and of itself, leads you to more happiness. Keep working on it!" – The Dalai Lama

Super Power Deep Breathing:
Secret of Endurance, Stamina & Longevity

How well your lungs function may predict how long you live. No doubt you have noticed rosy-cheeked children playing – running, jumping rope, skating and bicycling. They inhale large amounts of oxygen while doing these activities, and this we must keep in mind. We must keep active! We must exercise and take long, brisk walks and cultivate deep breathing. When people live sedentary lives and no longer get vigorous exercise, they are harming themselves and shortening their lives. Framingham Heart Studies showed the importance of how well you breathe is to a healthy lifestyle and longevity. *FraminghamHeartStudy.org.*

We had a long-time friend named Amos Stagg who was a famous California football and athletic coach. He lived over 100 active, healthy years! We asked him his secret of long life at his 100th birthday party. His answer was, *"I have the greater part of my life indulged in running and vigorous exercise that forced large amounts of oxygen into my body and along with working with athletes, has kept me youthful and interested in staying healthy, fit and alive!"*

Dad had a friend in New York, James Hocking, who was one of the greatest long-distance walking champions this country has ever had. We asked him on his 100th birthday the secret of his long, active, super healthy life. His answer, *"I have always walked vigorously and breathed deeply."* Oxygen is a cleansing detoxifier like fasting. His daily deep breathing helped cleanse the toxins from his body.

Dad and I have practiced deep breathing and believe people should expose their bodies to free currents of moving air. Air baths are important for good health! Whenever possible sleep with your windows wide open with cross ventilated air moving across your body. You sleep better and have a deeper night's rest if you wear light sleeping garments of cotton or silk – or nothing at all. You will be warm under the covers. But if you sleep with heavy blankets and nightwear, you smother your skin's vital oxygen supply and increase your chance of illness.

Healthy Walking Helps Solve Problems

You will find you can solve most problems on a brisk one to three mile walk. Whenever we have a problem to solve, we take a long brisk walk in the fresh air and even in the rain (Bragg follower Conrad Hilton walked rain or shine). By the time we finished our walk, we usually found a solution! We believe everyone should enjoy taking brisk short walks (arms swinging) an hour after their evening meal – even if it is up and down their driveway. Today people have become sitters. They sit at their work, movies, concerts, sport events, and in front of the T.V., and their computers at home. They are starved for more oxygen, exercise and circulation!

You must compensate for the hours you spend sitting down, because it inhibits your circulation and natural, healthy breathing! If your work and lifestyle require a lot of sitting, you should compensate for it with outdoor brisk walking and more vigorous physical activities daily. When you cannot get the carbon dioxide out of your body, you develop aches, pains and become prone to premature ageing! This is due to a lack of physical activity and sufficient oxygen. On city streets, you can see pale, ghostly people, unhealthy and exhausted – perhaps as a result of oxygen-starvation and poor lifestyle choices!

It's critical to fast, because it enables you to clean out some of this concentrated, stored-up carbon dioxide that failed to leave your body by deep breathing. When you are fasting, enjoy walking – even if it is a short walk. Make it a regular part of your life to be an active person! This doesn't mean house walks. It means getting out in the fresh air and having brisk walks, hiking, biking, running, tennis, swimming or dancing, etc. You must not allow any carbon dioxide to build up in your body – it will bring on health problems!

Make it a point every day of your life to breathe deeply during a vigorous brisk walk or some other aerobic exercise. Take long, slow, deep breaths every time you think of it. Soon your slow, deep breathing becomes a normal habit. When you combine deep breathing with fasting and living The Bragg Healthy Lifestyle, you are building more health, energy and vitality! Remind yourself daily *Doctor Fresh Air is your very important constant friend!*

173

HEALTHY HEART HABITS FOR LONG, VITAL LIFE

Remember, *organic live foods make live people. You are what you eat, drink, breathe, think, say and do.* So eat a low-fat, low-sugar, high-fiber diet of organic fresh raw salads, sprouts, greens, vegetables, whole grains, fruits, raw seeds, nuts, fresh juices and chemical-free, purified or distilled water.

Earn your food with daily exercise. For regular exercise, brisk walking, improves your health, stamina, go-power, flexibility, endurance and helps open the cardiovascular system! Only 45 minutes a day truly can do miracles for your heart, arteries, mind, nerves, soul and body! You become revitalized with new zest for living to accomplish your life goals!

We are made of tubes. To help keep them open, clean and to maintain good elimination, I take 1 veg psyllium cap or add 1 tsp psyllium husk powder daily an hour after dinner to juices, herbal teas, even apple cider vinegar drink. I also take one Cayenne capsule (40,000 HU) daily with a meal. I take 50 to 100 mgs. regular-released Niacin (B3) with one meal daily to help cleanse and open the cardiovascular system; also improves memory. Skin flushing may occur, don't worry about this as it shows it's working! After cholesterol level reaches 180, then only take Niacin twice weekly.

The heart needs healthy balanced nutrients, so take natural multi-vitamin-mineral food supplements: Omega-3 and extra heart helpers – vitamin E with mixed tocotrienols; vitamin C; Ubiquinol CoQ10; vitamin D3; MSM; D-Ribose; garlic; turmeric; selenium; zinc; beta carotene and amino acids – L-Carnitine, L-Taurine, L-Lysine and Proline. Folic acid, CoQ10, vitamin B6 and B12 helps keep homocysteine level low. Magnesium orotate, hawthorn berry extract helps bring relief for palpitations, arrhythmia, senile hearts and coronary disease. Take multi-digestive enzyme and probiotics with meals; it aids in digestion, assimilation and elimination.

174

For sleep problems try 5-HTP tryptophan (an amino acid), melatonin, calcium, magnesium, valerian (in capsule, extract or tea), and Sleepytime herb tea. For arthritis or joint pain/stiffness, try aloe juice or gel, glucosamine-chondroitin-MSM combo caps and shots, helps heal and regenerate. Capsaicin and DMSO lotion helps relieve pain. Natural liver cleanses to repair and regenerate include: milk thistle; dandelion root; artichoke and turmeric. Dandelion root is a natural diuretic and helps clear toxins through urination and also helps stimulate liver bile flow so waste can be eliminated.

Use amazing antioxidants – E Tocotrienols, vitamin C, quercetin, grape seed extract (OPCs), CoQ10, selenium, SOD, resveratrol, and alpha-lipoic acid. They improve immune system and help flush out dangerous free radicals that cause havoc with cardiovascular pipes and health. Research shows antioxidants promote longevity, slow ageing, fight toxins, help prevent disease, cancer, cataracts and exhaustion.

Recommended Heart Health Tests (for Adults):

- **Total Cholesterol:** 180 mg/dl or less is optimal
- **LDL Cholesterol:** 130 mg/dl or less is optimal • **HDL Cholesterol:** 50 mg/dl or more
- **Triglycerides:** 150 mg/dl or less is normal level
- **HDL/Cholesterol Ratio:** 5.0 or less • **Triglycerides/HDL Ratio:** below 2
- **Homocysteine:** 6-9 micromoles/L
- **CRP (C-Reactive Protein high sensitivity):**
  - • 1 mg/L = low risk • 1-3 mg/L = average risk • over 3 mg/L = high risk
- **Diabetic Risk Tests:**
  - **Glucose:** (do 12 hour food fast) 80-100 mg/dl • **Hemoglobin A1c:** 6% or less
- **Blood Pressure:** 120/70 mmHg is good for adults

Chapter 22

Doctor Exercise

Activity is Life, Stagnation is Death

Doctor Exercise makes this assertion . . . *To be lazy is to rust and rust means decay and destruction!* If we don't use our muscles, they loose their tone and life! To keep muscles firm, strong and youthful, they must be continually used! **Activity is the Law of Health and Life! Action is the Law of Well-Being!** All of the body's vital organs have specific functions that depend upon health and strength. Regular exercise helps to maintain and normalize weight, blood pressure, blood sugar and your cholesterol and fat levels.

When we exercise, we increase our physical strength, stamina, suppleness and good circulation! Daily exercise improves digestion, elimination and strengthens the muscles, especially the heart! If we are lazy and don't use our 640 muscles, our circulation, muscles and health all suffer from lack of exercise! The unused muscles become flabby, weak, unhealthy and unable to sustain active exercise.

175

Regular Exercise Promotes Healthy Skin & Body

People who exercise regularly are happier and have healthier, firmer skin tone. When we exercise, we bring on healthy perspiration from our body's 96 million pores. (Health Clubs have steam/ sauna rooms to enjoy that open your pores.) Skin is the body's largest eliminative organ (often called your third kidney). If someone gilded your body, clogging all your pores, you would die within minutes.

When you are exercising and perspiring freely, impurities and toxic poisons are being expelled. This allows the skin to perform its natural function of eliminating these poisons. If you don't exercise daily to the point of some perspiration, the cleansing work that the pores should be doing can throw a burden on the other eliminative organs and then some physical troubles can occur.

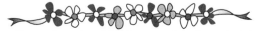

If you don't use it, you lose it – it's also true for the mind, body and spirit.

Enjoy Heart Healthy Exercise

Vigorous exercise helps to normalize blood pressure and helps create a healthier pulse. Vigorous exercise acts as an anticoagulant, which means it helps keep the blood from forming the clots which can cause a heart attack or stroke. **Daily exercise and brisk walking works miracles!**

Exercise Promotes Healthy Elimination

Every creature and human eliminates internal waste by means of muscular action. Inside your intestinal tract, there are three muscular layers which undergo a precise rhythmic, *wavelike-squeeze-push* called peristalsis. If you allow the internal and external abdominal muscles (important for elimination) to become inactive, flabby and fat instead of muscular, they lose their power to contract normally. The results: intestinal clogging which can cause constipation and even some diarrhea at times.

What happens when stomach muscles become weak and infiltrated with fat? They often refuse to work regularly. Then intestinal waste that should have been eliminated piles up. Fecal and toxic waste build-ups cause ill health. This sluggish inactivity can cause many serious diseases.

The Importance of Abdominal Exercises

The most important exercises stimulate all muscles of the human trunk from hips to armpits. These are the binding muscles which hold all vital organs in place. In developing your torso muscles, you are also developing vital muscles. As your back, waist, chest and abdomen increase in soundness and elasticity, so will your lungs, liver, heart, stomach and kidneys gain in efficiency and productivity. When exercising regularly, the arch of your ribs widens. This gives free play to lungs. Your elastic diaphragm allows the heart to pump and function more powerfully. Your rubberlike waist, in its limber action, stimulates the kidneys and massages the liver. Your abdominal muscles strengthen and support your stomach with controlled undulations. All this trunk exercise acts like a massage of vital organs and exerts an influence over the whole organism that must not be underestimated – as it is so vital for Super Health!

Exercise Relieves Varicose Veins, Ankle and Leg Swelling

If you sit or stand for a long time and your ankles become swollen, lie flat on your back, raise your legs and stretch your feet toward the ceiling and breathe deeply. You can also help to circulate any stagnant pooled blood (varicose veins) by using your hands to gently press downwards from ankles to hips. You will feel the blood flowing from your feet and ankles toward your heart. If you are in a place where you can't do this, breathe deeply in and out while you alternately rise up on your toes, then down and roll up on heels. Deep breathing and muscular action will stimulate circulation and help relieve the venous blood congestion and provide relief for aching legs and feet. These are good exercises upon awakening and before bedtime.

Enjoy Brisk Walks for Healthy Long Life

We recommend almost all forms of exercise, but feel daily brisk walking with arms swinging, is the best all-around exercise! This action of walking moves most of the body. Grasp the small of your back as you walk and feel how your entire frame responds to every stride and how the muscles work rhythmically. Walking promotes harmony of all the body's coordinating muscles. Your daily walk promotes healthier blood circulation, elimination, deeper breathing and helps normalize blood pressure, even diabetes and cholesterol.

Of all the many forms of exercise, brisk walking is the one that brings most of the body into action! It's the *king of exercise* and when the rhythm of your deep breathing and rhythm of your stride are in harmony, you feel more vibrant and alive! As the oxygen-filled blood courses through your body, your legs will carry you along buoyantly. Walk tall with your head held high, back straight, chest up, tummy in, arms swinging easily from your shoulders; legs moving as smoothly as though they were attached to the middle of your torso.

Our best preparation for tomorrow is the wise, proper use of today!

Brisk Walking is the King of Exercise

Walk briskly at least one to three miles every day and more when you have time. Don't make excuses! Make your daily walk a fixed routine no matter what kind of weather. In stormy weather, walk inside your home, on your porch or driveway, in the mall, etc. When traveling, use hotel hallways, stairs or even the treadmill or exercise equipment in the hotel's gym. **Walking can be done anytime, anywhere. Start today!**

We always preferred outdoor fresh air walking, but walking indoors is far better than no walking at all. When traveling the world on our Bragg Health Crusade tours, we often would take a light jog or a brisk evening walk through the corridors of our hotel or up and down the hotel stairs. Our favorite places for brisk walks are beaches, parks, hills and the open decks of cruise ships for the clean, fresh air.

Walking does not need to be done consciously. No heel and toe business. No getting there within a certain time limit. Let walking be as it is: the most functional of exercises. Carry yourself well. Walk naturally with your head high and chest up! You will feel physically elated and you will carry yourself proudly, straight and erect – yet relaxed and with an easy, smooth arm-swing. Vow to become a wonderful walker and make the day's walk a fixed item in your health program all the year round and in any kind of weather. Go at your own pace with your spirit free. If the outer world of Mother Nature fails to interest you, turn to the inner world of the mind. (Science says adults can grow new brain cells, see web: *salk.edu*)

In our opinion walking is better than golf. Life has so much to teach us that it's a time-waster trying to get a ball into a hole in a stroke less than another person. Unfortunately most golfers now use electric golf carts which eliminates the best part of golf – walking!

178

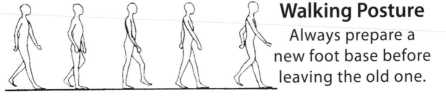

Walking Posture
Always prepare a new foot base before leaving the old one.

Miracle–Walking Builds New Blood Vessels

American Health reported that Dr. Gary Giangola, a vascular surgeon at New York University Medical Center, prescribed walking instead of bypass surgery for one of his patient's atherosclerosis. It was so pervasive it had severely restricted the blood flow to the legs and was causing extreme pain and numbness in his patient's feet. Dr. Giangola told his patient that if he walked one mile every day (even if he had to stop every two blocks to rest and recover), it would help build new blood vessels (collaterals) which would help bypass his closed arteries. He enjoyed his recovery! One year later the patient was able to enjoy walking several miles every day. Start walking!

Organic Gardening is Fun – Plus Exercise

Gardening is a marvelous form of exercise. It gives you exercise in the open air to help keep you more flexible. But you can gain weight even if you garden because there is too little movement. Achieve your goals by applying your energy productively in your organic vegetable and flower gardens, then take the kink out of your back with a healthy brisk walk and stretching! Personally, we've enjoyed combining these: swimming, tennis, biking, calisthenics, hiking and brisk walking. We love walking. We also love garden exercise. Find your favorite exercise combinations.

As a single footstep will not make a path on the earth, so a single thought will not make a pathway in the mind. To make a deep physical path, we walk again and again! To make a deep mental path, we must think over and over the kind of wise thoughts we wish to dominate our lives.
– Henry D. Thoreau

Make fitness a lifestyle with a Flex™ Heart Monitor – WIRELESS ACTIVITY and SLEEP WRISTBAND. This wristband device keeps track of your walking distance and even calories burned. If worn at night, it tracks sleep quality and wakes you silently in the morning. It's the motivation you need to get walking and be more active! – fitbit.com

Cold Water Swimmers are Fit and Ageless

My father prided himself on being able to endure the coldest weather wearing only a small amount of clothing, and he also enjoyed swimming in all parts of the world, in all kinds of weather. He was well known for his cold water swimming and welcomed as a member at Polar Bear Clubs worldwide. On many occasions, Dad and famous pioneer Dr. Robert Jackson had great

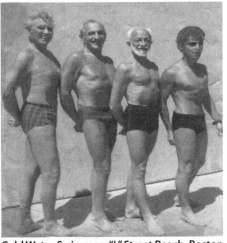

Cold Water Swimmers "L" Street Beach, Boston
Paul C. Bragg and Dr. John H. Federkiewicz,
David Cooper and Dr. David Carmos (the youngest)

sport breaking the ice and swimming with the amazing Boston Brownies of the famous "L" Street Bath House in Massachusetts. Here one could find some of the finest ageless physical specimens in the world, including people in their 60's, 70's, 80's 90's, and even over 100 years.

The same is true of the Polar Bears of Coney Island and at Montrose Beach in Chicago and those at the popular Bradford Beach in Milwaukee, Wisconsin. These healthy, hearty people who enjoy swimming in ice-cold water are all deep, full breathers. Many of them follow our Bragg System of Super Power Breathing. When you Super Power Breathe, you may also enjoy cold water swimming because both deep breathing and swimming are very invigorating and energizing!

We certainly don't recommend that everyone jump into ice-cold water! Let's leave that to people who have developed bodies with perfect thermostatic control. You can start slowly with alternating cold and warm showers. These swimmers are just examples of the power your body can develop when you are filled with oxygen at all times. There is no limit to your powers of resistance or your feeling of well-being when every cell in your body is filled with precious life-giving oxygen!

Studies show that athletes tend to have higher HDL (good cholesterol) levels.

180

Opera and Broadway Singers, Ballet Dancers and Champion Athletes are Deep Breathers

Breath control, by deep diaphragmatic breathing, is vital for all professional singers. Without the benefit of loudspeakers, the voices of the early great opera singers filled the auditoriums of the Metropolitan, La Scala and other famous opera houses throughout the world. What diaphragms they had! Look at the builds of these men and women. They have beautiful, perfect posture; superior development of the torso and tremendous lung capacity. Listen to the great recorded classic voices of Enrico Caruso and Mario Lanza, and those of other tenors who have thrilled the world, such as Luciano Pavarotti, Plácido Domingo and José Carreras. Hear their perfect voice control, from the softest pure note to the swell of a great crescendo. Study the lives of these extraordinary people and you will find that, regardless of their age, their attention to health and deep breathing filled them with energy and vitality.

Secret of Hollywood's Dancing Greats: Diaphragmatic Breathing

The same is true of all great dancers. The famous Ruth St. Denis and Ted Shawn, thrilled audiences throughout their long lifetimes, from their teens into their 70's. Deep diaphragmatic breathing was key to the tremendous energy and muscular control they brought to their spectacular dances! It was also key to their long, healthy, vibrant lives filled with super energy.

Deep diaphragmatic breathing is a basic component of the rigorous training of all the famous ballet companies. Many of Hollywood's great dancers like Fred Astaire, Gene Kelly, Arthur Murray and rollicking Rockettes of New York's Radio City Music Hall were living The Bragg Healthy Lifestyle. In order to have super energy, dancers find it to be important to live a healthy lifestyle and as a result, many live long lives, maintaining perpetual youthfulness.

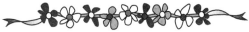

Age does not depend upon years, but upon lifestyle and health!

The beauty, strength, energy and endurance of dancers amaze us. Their secret is the excellent development of diaphragm breathing. Because their lungs draw in and expel large quantities of fresh air, they often have exquisite skin tone and flawless complexions, sparkling eyes, plus remarkably graceful and supple bodies.

Even if you aren't a singer or dancer, there is no reason why you shouldn't also enjoy good health and a long, happy, productive life. Without having to undergo the rigorous training of a professional performer, you can profit from their key secrets: deep diaphragmatic breathing, regular exercise, a healthy lifestyle and a natural diet.

Should We Exercise During Fasting?

Only the faster can answer this question. If there is no inclination for physical activity during a fast, then don't exercise. At most do some relaxing stretches and deep breathing! The fast is giving you a physiological rest. Unless you have a big urge for physical activity, you should relax and rest as much as possible when fasting.

 During a fast, your body is using all of its Vital Force for internal purification. But if during a 7 to 10 day fast you feel the need for some stretching or walking, respond to the urge. It's between fasts and in your daily program of living that you should spend a portion of every day of your life exercising, preferably outdoors. Soon you will enjoy a more vigorous circulation instead of a sluggish one. Poor body circulation causes many health problems, discomfort and pain throughout the body.

Fasting & Exercise Promotes Health & Energy

Fasting and a healthy lifestyle are your friends in your pursuit of youthfulness, health and balance. When it comes to fighting fat – diet and fasting come first! When it comes to keeping fit, exercise matters most. They all help each other; by enjoying daily exercise you may be more generous with your diet and your body machine should work better and enjoy more efficiency! All machines improve with wise, intelligent use. Nothing

Fasting is cleansing, purifying and restful. – Meir Schneider, Ph.D., founder of Meir Schneider's School for Self Healing and author of "Miracle Eyesight Method"

betrays a machine's weak areas as much as inactivity, and lack of regular maintenance and the inadequate, low-energy fuel! For example: your car needs routine maintenance, including gas, oil changes, tune-ups, etc.

The more you fast, the more toxins you cleanse from your body! As your body increases its internal cleanliness, your muscles will enjoy more energy, tone and vitality. You will find that your old, sluggish, lazy feelings will leave you and you will then desire more action and more physical activity! Life will become more exciting! When people don't exercise, their ankles and legs often swell because there's not enough blood circulating to remove the waste from the cells and carry it back to the organs of elimination! Allow no excuses for not exercising! Regardless of your physical condition, it's vitally important that some form of exercise become a part of your Healthy Lifestyle! Plot out a plan and get started now!

Exercise Helps Avert Sickness and Ageing!

Exercise helps builds a health fund of endurance and resistance! It helps build a healthy bloodstream with balanced white and red corpuscles that help keep us healthy by keeping our immune system on constant guard to fight off any germs, illnesses, etc. Exercise helps maintain a serene and tranquil mind and increases confidence. A one to three mile brisk walk in the fresh air helps neutralize most all unhealthful emotional upsets! The knowledge that you have improved your mental and physical abilities through exercise will give you supreme confidence. Exercise helps cultivate willpower and gives you control of your Physical, Mental and Spiritual Self which helps you to further promote your personal efficiency, happiness and longevity!

Exercise is the greatest health tonic we can provide ourselves! To attain this feeling of radiant, glorious health, follow The Bragg Healthy Lifestyle and engage in regular, vigorous physical activity. You will look and feel better and more youthful!

Exercise, deep breathing, healthy foods and fasting help maintain a healthier physical balance for a longer, happier life!

Stop Procrastinating – Start Exercising Daily

When it comes to these exercises – and in fact all exercises and habits of wise, healthy living – what is truly important is the DOING. "Knowing" and "wanting" are important too. But the "doing" is what it's all about. Don't play counter-productive games with yourself. The moment you begin asking yourself, "Do I have time to do this right now?" is the very moment to stop asking and start doing! The moment you begin to think, "I don't have the energy right now," is the very moment to stop thinking negatively and start doing. Be positive, start now! No more procrastinating!

Start the 10-Minute Trick – It Works Miracles

The successful students of The Bragg Healthy Lifestyle, and anyone who has successfully made healthy exercise part of their daily routine, will tell you the same thing: The moment of beginning is the most difficult. The in-between moment after you decide you want to become healthier and before you begin to act on that decision is the hardest moment. The moment before you put that one leg in front of the other on the first step of your brisk walk is the most difficult moment of the exercise.

The people who tell the success stories of exercise recommend "tricking yourself" into exercising at first. Play the "10 minute trick." Before you start (the hardest moment), tell yourself, "I'll only exercise, walk, etc. for 10 minutes and then I'll stop. That will be easy and I'll be done soon." Once you've done this, you're on the path to healthy fitness – and it will be fun! Once this most difficult moment is over (the beginning) you'll find when the 10 minute mark comes around you are enjoying yourself too much to quit so soon!

184

It's Never Too Late to Start Exercising

Studies show it's never too late to begin exercising. Recent physical activity has a greater positive impact on cardiovascular disease and mortality than exercise done in one's past. The cardiovascular health benefits of recent physical activity are more pronounced than with distant physical activity, even though both are beneficial. A consistent maintenance exercise program produced the best overall results!
– Sports Medicine Digest • www.TheSportDigest.com

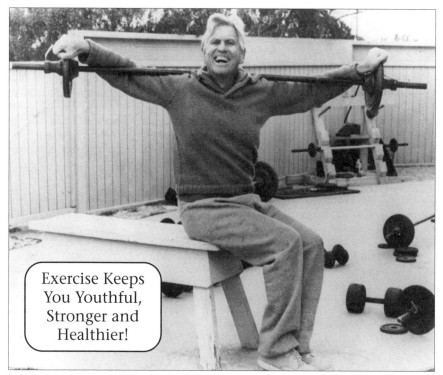

Exercise Keeps You Youthful, Stronger and Healthier!

Paul and Patricia enjoyed lifting weights three times weekly.

Building Up a Healthy Body with Exercise

Exercise helps to normalize blood pressure and create a healthy pulse. It keeps the blood flowing smoothly and not clotting. Staying active keeps you feeling energized!

Studies have proven that weight-lifting rejuvenates oldsters. Demonstrating it is never too late to reverse an age-related decline in muscle strength and shows the great importance of keeping the 640 muscles as active and fit as possible to maintain general overall good health! Try it – it has worked for us and others! One study concluded: "A three-days-a-week weight-training program is capable of inducing a dramatic increase in health, longevity and muscle strength in frail men and women even up to 96 years of age."

Staying active is like riding an UP elevator. The more you do, the more you feel like staying involved. Even couch potatoes can become active and fit!

If exercise could be packed into a pill, it would be the single most widely prescribed and beneficial medicine in America. – Robert Butler, M.D.

Do These Exercises Daily (10 per set):

Exercise is a must! It is of the utmost importance because weak muscles of the arms, legs and entire body indicate a similar unhealthy condition of the stomach muscles, heart and other vital important body organs.

> **Important Exercises for Keeping External and Internal Muscles of The Stomach and Back Fit and Healthy. These Also Promote Good Elimination and Energy.**

Bend at the waist to the sides, then front and back.

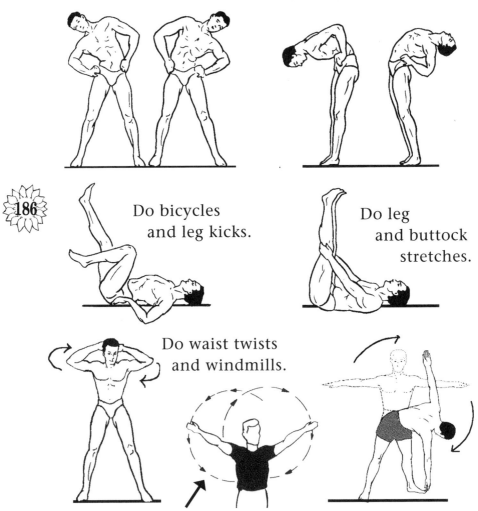

186

Do bicycles and leg kicks.

Do leg and buttock stretches.

Do waist twists and windmills.

WINDMILL EXERCISE: Swing arms forward and go around in large circles. Let your hands feel heavy and let the hands carry your arms around and around. Now do backward circles. Breathe easily and deeply, feet 12" apart, bend knees a little and then straighten them up with each circle. Do 3 to 5 times daily. Results: tension goes, energy increases!

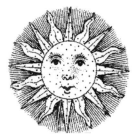

Chapter 23

Doctor Gentle Sunshine

Doctor Sunshine's specialty is heliotherapy and the most popular prescription is solar energy! Each blade of grass, every vine, tree, bush, flower, fruit and vegetable draws its life from solar energy. All living things on earth depend on solar energy for their existence. The earth would be a barren, frigid place if it were not for the magic sun rays! The sun gives us light, and were it not for light, there would be no you or me! Earth would be in total darkness and void of life.

A person's skin is gently tanned by the sun and air and will take on a darker pigment according to its original skin tone. It has been found that with gentle exposure to the sun even redheaded people will eventually tan. Pigmentation is a sign that solar energy has been **187** transformed into human energy. Mankind can gain health and vitality in the gentle, healing rays of the sun (page 189).

The rays of the sun are powerful germicides! As the skin imbibes more of these rays, it stores up enormous amounts of this germ-killing energy. The gentle sun provides a remedy for the nervous person filled with anxiety, worry, stresses and strains. When these tense people lie in the early morning or late afternoon gentle sunshine, its healing rays give them what the nerves and body are crying out for . . . and that is gentle relaxation!

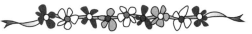

Freedom and progress rest in man's continual searching for truth.
Truth is the summit of being. – Ralph Waldo Emerson

There is no substitute for Good Health!
Those who possess health are richer than kings! – Paul C. Bragg, N.D., Ph.D.

What sculpture is to a block of marble, education is to the mind and soul.
– Joseph Addison, "The Spectator Newspaper," England, 1711

Chlorophyll is Miracle Liquid Sunshine

Gentle sunshine is a soothing tonic, a stimulant and above all, the Great Healer! As you bask in the warm, gentle sunshine (not the hot afternoon sun), millions of nerve endings absorb the energy from the sun and transform it so the body's nervous system can use it.

Perform this experiment to determine the value of sunshine in the matter of life and death. Find a beautiful lawn, where the grass is like a green carpet. Cover up a small space of that beautiful lawn with a piece of wood or a small box. Day by day you will soon notice that the beautiful grass that once was full of plant blood, precious chlorophyll, will fade and turn a sickly yellow. Tragically, it withers and dies – death by sun starvation! The same thing happens in your body without the sun's life-giving rays and without an abundance of sun-ripened foods such as organic fruits, vegetables and their fresh juices.

We must have the direct gentle rays of the sun on our bodies and at least 60% to 70% percent of the food we eat ripened by the sun's rays. When we eat fresh, organically grown fruits and vegetables, we absorb the blood of the plant – chlorophyll. This life-giving chlorophyll is the solar energy that the plant has absorbed from the sun, the richest, most nourishing health food you can put in your body. Green plants and vegetables alone possess the secret of how to capture this powerful solar energy and pass it on to man and every other living creature. When you absorb sunshine on the outside of your body and eat ample sun-grown, organic fruits and vegetables, you are going to glow with more super health! But this powerful, natural remedy must be taken in small doses at the beginning, because your sun-starved body can't absorb too much at first.

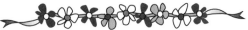

God gave His creatures light and air and water open to the skies;
Man locks himself in a stifling lair and wonders why his brother dies.
– Oliver W. Holmes, Associate Justice to U.S. Supreme Court, 1902-1932

Nature never deceives us; it's always we who deceive ourselves. – Rousseau

---

Let your inner light happily shine brightly. – Beatrex Quntanna

Gentle Sunbathing Works Miracles!

When you begin sunbathing, start with short time periods until you condition your body to take more. The best time for beginners to start taking 10 and 15 minute sunbaths is in the early morning sunshine until 10 a.m. or late afternoon sunshine after 3 p.m. Between 11 and 3 we usually avoid stronger, burning rays.

The same caution should be taken when eating sun-ripened raw fruits and vegetables. The average person who has been eating mainly cooked foods will find that if great amounts of raw fruits and vegetables suddenly enter into the body they can cause a reaction. It's wiser to gradually add more sun-ripened foods to the diet. Overdoses of solar energy, both outside and inside the body, are not wise. Regarding sun exposure, use good judgment and caution. For sun (skin) protection make a green herb tea, then bottle, apply to skin when needed.

Doctor Healing Sunshine Saved Bragg's Life!

When my father was diagnosed with tuberculosis at 16, three TB Sanitariums later, the best TB doctors in USA declared his case *hopeless and incurable!* Yet, by the grace of God, he was led to Dr. August Rollier of Leysin, Switzerland, the greatest living authority on heliotherapy (sun cure). High in the Swiss Alps, Dad's sick and wasted body was exposed to the gentle healing rays of the sun and was fed an abundance of natural, sun-ripened foods.

A healing miracle happened. In just two years he was transformed from a hopeless invalid to a vitally strong young man who radiated health! Throughout Paul Bragg's long, fulfilled life he was healthy, happy, powerful in sports and always enjoyed the great outdoors and the healing rays of the gentle sun on his body.

 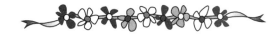

Laughter is a sunbeam for the soul.
– Thomas Mann, author, "The Magic Mountain"

Wherever you go, no matter what the weather,
always bring your own sunshine. – Anthony J. D'Angelo

189

Paul C. Bragg Found Peace, Relaxation and Joy – and then Crusaded to Share it with the World!

Many people talk about relaxing – just as I used to talk about it. But only after years of consistent healthy lifestyle living with fasting and purification did I really learn to completely relax! Each day I'm able to release all tensions from my nerves and muscles and thus renew my vitality and energy through complete relaxation. I sleep better now than I did when I was a child! I find that no matter where I am – no matter what the noise or excitement may be – I can sit or lie down, close my eyes and completely relax. This I want for you also!

*I find I'm able to understand other people now when they become upset and emotional. I'm therefore better able to help them calm down. I feel I'm growing – and not only on the physical side! I believe I'm not only building a powerful physical body but, through cleansing and fasting, I'm also advancing mentally and spiritually. I constantly search for light, truth and education along all lines. I find I have a greater interest in everything that is happening in the world. I find I understand people better and in understanding others, I'm able to better understand myself. This way of life opens many doors that lead to higher life! After all, as we journey through life we should grow and balance our lives physically, mentally, emotionally and spiritually. Many of our worldwide health followers write us about this newly discovered strength in mental and spiritual growth they are experiencing. They rejoice when they have found peace in their mind, soul and total being. **This is the true joy of healthy living!***

I'm a happy man! I have no worries, no fears and no false ambitions! I lead a simple, healthy, happy fulfilled life and give thanks for all my blessings daily! **with love,**
Remember Patricia and I are your health friends for eternity. *Paul C. Bragg*

Dear friend, I wish above all things that thou may prosper and be in health even as the soul prospers. – 3 John 2

Nothing in all creation is so like God as soothing stillness. – Meister Eckhart

Chapter 24

Healthy Alternatives to Help with Breathing Problems
• Nutritional, Herbal & Water Therapy
• Massage • Acupuncture • Chiropractic
• Natural Alternative Therapies

Don't Accept Breathing Problems – Solve Them

The healthiest, best thing to do instead of taking drugs for asthma, sinus, bronchitis, COPD and other breathing problems is to seek natural remedies to correct any problems! Drugs should never be the main method of seeking a cure. These drugs and applications are commonly called "maintenance drugs." Even this is misleading because the problems they supposedly relieve often get worse over time, not to mention the many other side effects they have on the entire body!

191

The three prominent types of drugs for sinus and asthma problems are: bronchodilators (see pages 81-85) anti-inflammatories and antihistamines. Although the first two can supply some relief during attacks by opening narrowed breathing pathways, they can be dangerous and ill-advised. A study of bronchodilators, (drug puffers) in New Zealand found that their habit forming use brought an increased risk of asthma-related deaths and injury. Antihistamines, on the other hand, really promise no relief to asthma sufferers, even in the short-term. Their effect is merely to dry up mucus secretions and replace the aggravating plugs of thick mucus with dried, clogging crusts of mucus.

For a healthy nose, it's essential to live The Bragg Healthy Lifestyle. Practice this lifestyle formula for good physical and mental health! A healthy head and body are necessary preconditions to a healthy, happy nose (see pages 33-39)!

According to medical studies more people suffer from a condition called multiple chemical sensitivity. Now it is more crucial that you and your family practice natural healthy living habits to stay healthy!

Pollution and Wrong Diet Affects Breathing

In addition, if you live in a polluted area, or if your sinuses are already damaged from the hard work of protecting your lungs, using a high-efficiency, charcoal particulate HEPA air filtration system can help. They pre-filter the air your sinuses will filter, making your nose's job easier. Have one for your home, office and car (see page 115).

You must also be intelligent about your allergies. If you know you are allergic to particular substances, take precautions to avoid them. If you suspect allergies, take the necessary steps to learn what's affecting you. The most common allergens are mold spores, animal hair and dander, toxic house dust, mites, pollens and even carpet and paint chemicals, etc. Food allergies are also a frequent source of allergic respiratory reactions (see page 37-38).

With long-term relief in mind, stay informed about the effective alternative therapies available today. The most sensible therapy to practice, no matter what the health complaint, is **Nutritional Therapy**. When it comes to sinus problems it's most important to avoid dairy products of all kinds. Dairy foods are unhealthy for the nose and the whole body. Dairy proteins often mimic allergens by causing the nose and throat airway passages to swell. They also increase mucus production. This in turn causes sinus discomfort and can give rise to dangerous bacterial conditions. If you are a snorer (see page 95-97) or a sufferer of any sinus condition you will especially benefit from a no-dairy diet. Try it – prove it to yourself!

In addition to healthy living and avoiding all dairy, you can relieve sinusitis symptoms and bolster the health of your nose by using **Herbal Therapy** such as: licorice, anise and horehound, Brigham tea, mint, echinacea, fenugreek, goldenseal, lobelia, marshmallow, mullein, red clover and rose hips (see page 36). Herbs are available in teas, capsules or tablets. Medicinal herbs, soaked in a cloth poultice (hot), can provide relief for sore, congested areas. (Example: old fashion mustard chest pack for chest colds.)

192

The Lord gives strength to those who are weary. – Isaiah 40:29

Perfect health is above gold; a sound body before riches. – Solomon

No matter what therapies you practice, consider *Water Therapy*, a health essential! Never fail to drink at least 8 tall glasses of purified/distilled water daily. This helps your mucus membranes and sinuses efficiently filter and dispose of any contaminants that you breathe in the air. In this book we have continued to inform you of all the various health alternatives for your health!

Also try this soothing detox shower: apply olive oil to skin, alternate hot and cold water, every 2-3 minutes. Massage body while under hot, filtered spray. Garden hose massage is great in summer. Try a hot detox soaking bath (diabetics use warm water) for 20 minutes with one cup of Epsom salts. This soak helps pull out toxins by creating an artificial fever cleanse.

Healthy Alternative Massage Techniques

REIKI: A Japanese form of massage that means "Universal Life Energy." Reiki Massage helps the body to detoxify, then re-balance and heal itself. Discovered in the ancient Sutra manuscripts by Dr. Mikao Usui in Japan 1922. Web: *Reiki.org*

ROLFING: Developed by Ida Rolf in the 1930's in the U.S. Rolfing is also called structural processing and postural release, or structural dynamics. It is based on the concept that distortions (accidents, injuries, falls, etc.) and the effects of gravity on the body cause upsets and long-term stress in the body. Rolfing helps to achieve balance and improved body posture. Methods involve the use of stretching, with gentle deep tissue massage and relaxation techniques to loosen old injuries, break bad movement and posture patterns. Web: *Rolf.org*

TRAGERING: Founded by Dr. Milton Trager M.D., who was inspired at age 18 by Paul C. Bragg to become a doctor. It is a mind-body learning method that involves gentle shaking and rocking, allowing the body to let go, releasing tensions and lengthening the muscles for more body peace and health. Tragering can do miracle healing where needed in the body frame, muscles and the entire body. Web: *Trager.com*

Time waits for no one, treasure and protect every moment you have!

MASSAGE & AROMATHERAPY: works two ways: the essence (aroma) relaxes, as does healing massage. Essential oils are extracted from flowers, leaves, roots, seeds and barks. These are usually massaged into skin, inhaled or used in a bath to help the body relax, soothe and heal. The oils, used for centuries to treat numerous ailments, are revitalizing and energizing for the body and mind. Example: Tiger balm, MSM, echinacea and arnica help relieve muscle aches. (Avoid skin creams and lotions with mineral oil – it clogs the skin's pores.) Use these natural oils for the skin: almond, avocado, and organic olive oil and mix with aromatic essential oils: rosemary, lavender, rose, jasmine, sandalwood or lemon-balm, etc. – 6 oz. oil and 4 drops of an essential oil. Web: *www.Aromatherapy.com*

MASSAGE – SELF: Paul C. Bragg often said, *"You can be your own best massage therapist, even if you have only one good hand."* Near-miraculous health improvements have been achieved by victims of accidents or strokes in bringing life back to afflicted parts of their own bodies by self-massage and with vibrators. Treatments can be day or night, almost continual. Self-massage also helps achieve relaxation at day's end. Families and friends can learn and exchange massages; it's a wonderful sharing experience. Remember, babies love and thrive with daily massages, start from birth. Family pets also love soothing, healing touch of massages. Web: *RD.com/health/wellness/learn-the-art-of-self-massage*

194

MASSAGE – SHIATSU: Japanese massage form applies pressure from fingers, hands, elbows and even knees along the same points as acupuncture. Shiatsu originated in Japan and is based on traditional Chinese medicine, and has been widely practiced around the world since 1970s. Shiatsu has been used in Asia for centuries to relieve pain, common ills, muscle stress and to aid lymphatic circulation. See web: *centerpointmn.com/the-benefits-of-shiatsu-massage*

Caring hands have healing life-force energy . . . babies love and thrive with daily massages and cuddles. Family pets love soothing, healing touches. Everyone benefits from healing massages and treatments! – Patricia Bragg

 Where there is great love there are always miracles. – Willa Cather, Pulitzer Prize-winning author

MASSAGE – SPORTS: An important health support system for professional and amateur athletes. Sports massage improves circulation and mobility to injured tissue, enables athletes to recover more rapidly from myofascial injury, reduces muscle soreness and chronic strain patterns. Soft tissues are freed of trigger points and adhesions, thus contributing to improvement of peak neuromuscular functioning and athletic performance.

MASSAGE – SWEDISH: One of the oldest and the most popular and widely used massage techniques. This deep body massage soothes and promotes healthy circulation and is a great way to loosen and relax tight muscles before and after exercise. For more info see web: *www.MassageDen.com/swedish-massage.shtml*

Alternative Health Therapies for Healing Try Them – They Work Miracles!

Explore these wonderful natural methods of healing your body. Over 600 Medical Schools in the U.S. are teaching Healthy Alternative Therapies. Please check the websites. Seek and choose the best healing techniques for you: 195

ACUPUNCTURE / ACUPRESSURE: Acupuncture directs and rechannels body energy by inserting hair-thin needles (use only disposable needles) at specific points on the body. It's used for pain, backaches, migraines and general health and body dysfunctions. Used in Asia for centuries, acupuncture is safe, virtually painless and has no side effects! Acupressure is based on the same principles and uses finger pressure and massage rather than needles. Check web: *AcupunctureToday.com*

Author's Comment: We have personally sampled many of these Alternative Therapies. It's estimated America's health care costs are over $2.6 trillion. It's more important than ever to be responsible for our own health! This includes seeking dedicated holistic health practitioners to keep us well by inspiring us to practice prevention! These Alternative Healing Therapies are also popular and getting results: aromatherapy, Ayurvedic, biofeedback, color, guided imagery, herbs, hyperbaric oxygen, music, meditation, magnets, saunas, tai chi, Qi gong, Pilates, Rebounder, yoga, etc. Explore and be open to improving your earthly temple for a healthy, happier, longer life. Seek & find the best for your body, mind & soul. – Patricia Bragg

CHIROPRACTIC: was founded in Davenport, Iowa in 1885 by Daniel David Palmer. There are now many schools in the U.S., and graduates are joining Health Practitioners in all nations of the world to share healing techniques. Chiropractic is popular and the largest U.S. healing profession benefitting literally millions! Treatment involves soft tissue, spinal and body adjustment to free your nervous system of any interferences with normal body functions. Its concern is the functional integrity of the musculoskeletal system. In addition to manual methods, chiropractors use physical therapy modalities, exercise, health and nutritional guidance. Web: *ChiroWeb.com*

ALEXANDER TECHNIQUE: helps end improper use of neuromuscular system, helps bring body posture into balance. Eliminates psycho-physical interferences, helps release long-held tension, and aids in re-establishing muscle tone. For more info see web: *AlexanderTechnique.com*

FELDENKRAIS METHOD: Dr. Moshe Feldenkrais founded this in the late 1940s. This Method leads to improved posture and helps create ease and more efficiency of body movement. This Method is a great stress removal. Web: *Feldenkrais.com*

Healing Natural Therapy & Healthy Lifestyle

HOMEOPATHY: In 1796, Dr. Samuel Hahnemann, a German physician, developed homeopathy. Patients are treated with "micro" doses of remedies found in nature to trigger the body's own defenses. This homeopathic principle is a safe and nontoxic remedy and is the #1 alternative therapy in Europe and Britain because it is inexpensive, seldom has any side effects, and usually brings fast results. Web: *HomeopathyCenter.org*

NATUROPATHY: Brought to America by Dr. Benedict Lust, M.D., this treatment uses diet, herbs, homeopathy, fasting, exercise, hydrotherapy, manipulation and sunlight. Practitioners work with your body to restore health naturally. They reject surgery and drugs except as a last resort. Web: *www.Naturopathic.org*

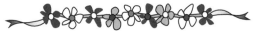

Harmful toxins enter the body through food, water, skin and air.

OSTEOPATHY: The first School of Osteopathy was founded in 1892 by Dr. Andrew Taylor Still, M.D. There are now 30 U.S. colleges. Treatment involves soft tissue, spinal and body adjustments that free the nervous system from interferences that can cause illness. Healing by adjustment also includes good nutrition, physical therapies, proper breathing and good posture. Dr. Still's premise: if the body structure is altered or abnormal, then proper body function is altered and can cause pain and illness. Web: *www.AcademyofOsteopathy.org*

REFLEXOLOGY / ZONE THERAPY: Founded by Eunice Ingham, author of *Stories The Feet Can Tell*, inspired by a Bragg Health Crusade when she was 17. Reflexology helps the body and organs by removing crystalline deposits from reflex areas (nerve endings) of feet and hands through deep pressure massage. Primitive reflexology originated in China and Egypt and Native American Indians and Kenyans self-practiced it for centuries. Reflexology activates your body's flow of healing and energy by dislodging deposits. Visit Eunice Ingham and nephew Dwight Byer's website: *www.Reflexology-usa.net*

COLON HYDROTHERAPY: is a safe and effective method for supporting detoxification, and improving health and vitality. Contact I-ACT (Int'l Association Colon Hydrotherapy) for a certified colon Hydro-Therapist in your area. Web: *i-act.org*

SKIN BRUSHING: daily is wonderful for circulation, toning, cleansing and healing. Use a dry vegetable brush (never nylon) and brush lightly. Helps purify lymph so it's able to detoxify your blood and tissues. Removes old skin cells, uric acid crystals and toxic wastes that come up through skin's pores. Use loofah sponge for variety in shower or tub.

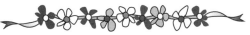

Perhaps the most valuable result of all education is the ability
to make yourself do the thing you have to do, when it ought to be done,
as it ought to be done, whether you like it or not!

Progress is impossible without change, and those who cannot
change their minds, cannot change anything.
– George Bernard Shaw

Health is Your Birthright –
Protect and Treasure It!

This is a priceless health book. Please read and re-read this book until you absorb every health nugget it contains. Remember that you and you alone control your life, your health and the way you look, act, think and feel! Health comes from the inside out. You can be patched up after being stricken with disease, sickness and physical pain, but 100% true, robust, vital health comes from good *health habits!* This book shows you how to turn away from damaging, unhealthy lifestyle habits that careless, improper living promotes in this hectic, fast-food age!

It is up to you to apply the intelligence. We teach simple, healthy living. You now have a treasure of knowledge of how to create a healthier, more joyful life through living this simple, healthy lifestyle. Have faith in yourself, start now!

Your health depends on how healthy your lifestyle is, the way you conduct yourself each hour, each day, each week, each month and each year! You are the sum total of your habits!

We have no supernatural power to prevent or cure disease. That power is in your body! Your body is self-cleansing and self-healing when given a chance. We can only come to you as health teachers, to tell you in a simple way what living this healthy lifestyle will do for you. **Living The Bragg Healthy Lifestyle is simply good common sense.**

Bragg Healthy Lifestyle Plan

- *Read, plan, plot, and follow through for supreme health and longevity.*

- *Underline, highlight or dog-ear pages as you read important passages.*

- *Organizing your lifestyle helps you identify what's important in your life.*

- *Be faithful to your health goals everyday for a healthy, long, happy life.*

- *Where space allows we have included "words of wisdom" from great minds to motivate and inspire you. Please share your favorite sayings with us.*

- *Please write us on your successes following The Bragg Healthy Lifestyle.*

Knowing these teachings will mean true life and good health for you.
– Proverbs 4:22

Earn Your Bragging Rights
Live The Bragg Healthy Lifestyle
To Attain Supreme Physical, Mental,
Emotional and Spiritual Health!

With your new awareness, understanding and sincere commitment of how to live The Bragg Healthy Lifestyle – you can now live a longer, healthier life to any age!

God bless you and your family!
With Blessings of Health, Peace, Joy and Love,

Paul and *Patricia*

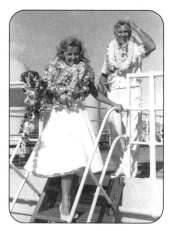

Health Crusaders Paul C. Bragg and daughter Patricia traveled the world spreading health, inspiring millions to renew and revitalize their health.

199

The Bragg books are written to inspire and guide you to health, fitness and longevity. Remember, the book you don't read won't help. So please reread Bragg Books and live The Bragg Healthy Lifestyle to enjoy a healthy fulfilled life!

I never suspected that I would have to learn how to live – that there were specific disciplines and ways of seeing the world that I had to master before I could awaken to a simple, healthy, happy, uncomplicated life. – Dan Millman, author "The Way of the Peaceful Warrior" • peacefulwarrior.com A Bragg fan and admirer since his Stanford University coaching days.

A truly good book teaches me better than to just read it, I must soon lay it down and commence living in its wisdom. What I began by reading, I must finish by acting! – Henry David Thoreau

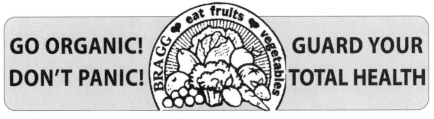

FROM THE AUTHORS

This book was written for You! It can be your passport to a healthy, long, vital life. We in the Alternative Health Therapies join hands in one common objective – promoting a high standard of health for everyone. Healthy nutrition points the way – which is Mother Nature's and God's Way. This book teaches you how to work with them, not against them! Health doctors, therapists, nurses, teachers and caregivers are becoming more dedicated than ever before to keeping their patients healthy and fit. This book was written to emphasize the great needed importance of healthy lifestyle living for health and longevity, close to Mother Nature and God.

Statements in this book are scientific health findings, known facts of physiology and biological therapeutics. Paul C. Bragg practiced natural methods of living for over 80 years with highly beneficial results, knowing they were safe and of great value. His daughter Patricia lectured and co-authored Bragg Health Books with him and continues carrying on The Bragg Healthy Lifestyle.

200

Paul C. Bragg and daughter Patricia express their opinions solely as Public Health Educators and Health Crusaders. They offer no cure for disease. Only the body has the ability to cure a person. Experts may disagree with some of the statements made in this book. However, such statements are considered to be factual, based on the long-time experience of dedicated pioneer Health Crusaders Paul C. Bragg and Patricia Bragg. If you suspect you have a medical problem, please always seek qualified Health Care professionals to help you make the healthiest, wisest and best-informed choices!

Count your blessings daily while you do your 30 to 45 minute brisk walks and exercises with these affirmations – health! strength! youth! vitality! peace! laughter! humility! understanding! forgiveness! joy! and love for eternity! and soon all these qualities will come flooding and bouncing into your life. With blessings of super health, peace and love to you, our dear friends – our readers. – Patricia Bragg, Health Crusader

If I were to name the three most precious resources of life, I would say books, friends and nature; and the greatest of these, at least the most constant and always at hand is Mother Nature and God. – John Burroughs

Praises and Testimonials for The Bragg Healthy Lifestyle

I regained my health by eating organic fruits and vegetables and taking supplements. I'm eating foods the way God created them and my body is thriving. Thanks for The Bragg Healthy Lifestyle – it's great!
– Candace Hawthorne, Metairie, Louisiana

Dr. Patricia Bragg is a dedicated Health Crusader and she shared her Bragg Healthy Lifestyle with millions of our TV and radio listeners. Thank you Patricia.
– Host George Noory • *www.CoastToCoastam.com*

I would like to thank you for teaching me how to take control of my health! I lost 55 pounds and I feel great! Bragg Health Books have showed me vitality, happiness and being close to Mother Nature. You both are real Health Crusaders for the World. Thanks. – Leonard Amato

---

Thanks to you and your wonderful father for your guidance and teaching over the years. What a great gift you and your father have provided for us all through your Bragg Health Books. Your Fasting and Vinegar books have improved my life immensely. I've lost 30 lbs. and feel years younger. At 67 youthful years, I give thanks for the great benefits of health I enjoy because of the work you and your father have so generously dedicated your lives too!! Wishing you every blessing under the Sun.
– Captain Wes Herman (retired)
Santa Barbara County Fire Dept.

I thank Paul Bragg for his Health Pioneering and Crusading. Dr. Bragg paved the way for our 100% healthy principles and inspired me to start the Good Earth Restaurants. – Bill Galt, CA

I give thanks to Health Crusaders Paul Bragg and daughter Patricia for their dedicated years of service spreading health as our Lord wants us healthy! It's made a great difference in my life and millions worldwide.
– Pat Robertson, Host CBN "700" Club

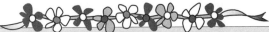

Praises and Testimonials for
The Bragg Healthy Lifestyle

I found your Bragg books from years ago. I have gotten off almost all my prescriptions drugs! Thanks for what you and your dad did for the health of millions. Forty years ago doctors didn't believe that food had anything to do with your health. Look where we are today. Your dad must be looking down from heaven seeing the footprints he made on the life of millions. God Bless. – Sharon

The Lord works sometimes in ways we don't expect. He chose to answer my prayer by leading me to your health books and way of living . . . thus my medical problems are GONE! I want to give thanks to God, and to you, Patricia and your father. It was the Bragg Health Books that converted me to Healthy Living . . . and I will never be the same again! Thank You and God Bless. – Jimmy Damianos, Florida

Thank you Patricia for our first meeting in London in 1968. When I was feeling my years, you gave me your *Miracle of Fasting* Book – it got me exercising – doing brisk walking and eating more wisely. You were a blessing God-sent and just when I needed to get more healthily recharged for Crusading. – Reverend Billy Graham • *www.BillyGraham.org*

In the past our family has had chronic health problems. Within the last year and a half God has shown us His will for healing and divine health. Our journey has included a healthy diet, some fasting and a complete change in lifestyle. I cannot express how good we feel! I am so thankful for every good thing that God has put before us – this journey, and every miraculous result and The Bragg Healthy Lifestyle is a part of that. Thank you for sharing this wealth of health in the Bragg Books. God Bless You! – Rhonda Jackson, Oklahoma

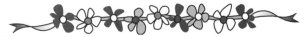

Exercise, along with healthy foods and some fasting helps maintain or restore a healthy physical balance and normal weight for a long happy life.

"You change your life by changing your heart." – Max Lucado

PATRICIA & PAUL C. BRAGG, N.D., Ph.D.
Dynamic Daughter & Father are World Health Crusaders

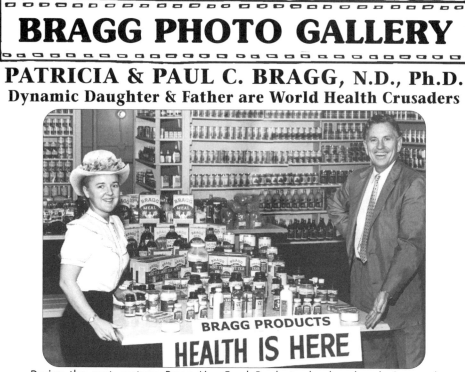

BRAGG PRODUCTS
HEALTH IS HERE

During the past century, Bragg Live Food Products developed and pioneered the very first line of Health Foods, from vitamins and minerals to organic nuts, seeds, and sun-dried fruits. This included over 365 health products, – *"one for each day of the year!"* says daughter Patricia Bragg.

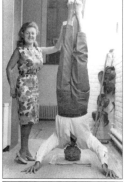

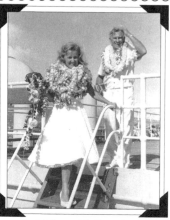

"Thanks for The Bragg Healthy Lifestyle that you shared with me and you are sharing with millions of others worldwide."
– John Gray, Ph.D., author

Picture from
People Magazine August, 1975.

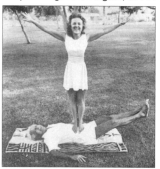

Patricia and father, Paul on world trip in 1950's, during stop in Tahiti.

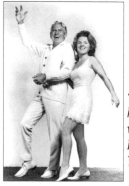

"You have recharged me with joy, hope, love and encouragement, which poured from your words. I am now fasting and using ACV. You have certainly improved my life!"
– Marie Furia, New Jersey

Patricia Bragg stands on her father's stomach. Paul's stomach muscles are so strong he can lift Patricia up and down!

203

PAUL C. BRAGG, N.D., Ph.D.
HEALTH CRUSADER
Life Extension Specialist and Originator of Health Food Stores

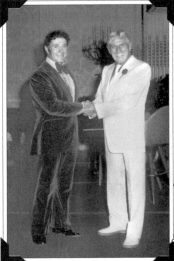

I have experienced a beautiful, remarkable, spiritual and physical awakening since reading Bragg Health Books. I'll never be the same again.
– Sandy Tuttle, Ohio

With every new day comes new strength and new thoughts.
– Eleanor Roosevelt

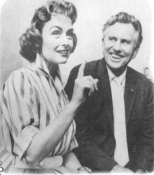

Actress Donna Reed saying "Health First" with Paul C. Bragg.

Dr. Paul C. Bragg (right) Creator Health Food Stores, Pioneer Life Extension Specialist, with his prize student Jack LaLanne. Paul started him on the royal road to health over 85 years ago!

Paul C. Bragg spent much of his time at the Hollywood Studios meeting with top Stars and motion picture industry executives, giving health lectures and private consultations. Dr. Paul C. Bragg was Hollywood's first highly respected, health, fitness and nutrition advisor to the Stars.

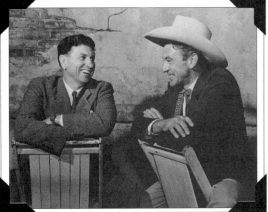

Paul C. Bragg with Gary Cooper, famous American film actor, best known for his many Western films.

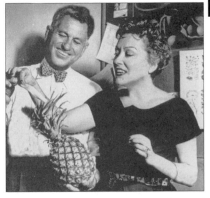

Paul C. Bragg with the famous Hollywood Actress Gloria Swanson, who was leading star in 20s, 30s and 40s. Gloria became a Bragg Health Devotee at 18 and she often would Health Crusade with Bragg during the 1950s.

204

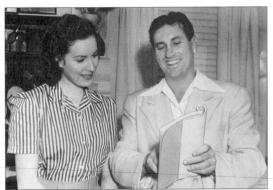

Maureen O'Hara and Paul C. Bragg. This Irish film actress and singer was best noted for playing in "Miracle on 34th Street" and "The Quiet Man."

PAUL C. BRAGG, N.D., Ph.D.
STAYING HEALTHY & FIT

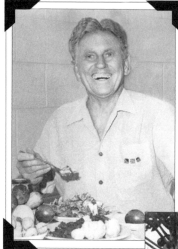

I'd like to thank you for teaching me how to take control of my health! I lost 55 pounds and I feel "great!" Bragg books have showed me vitality, happiness and being close to Mother Nature. You both are real "Crusaders for Health for the World." Thanks!
– Leonard Amato

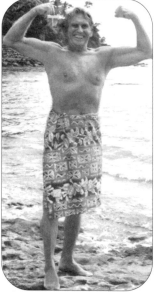

Dr. Paul C. Bragg and daughter Patricia were my early guiding inspiration to my health career.
– Jeffery Bland, Ph.D., Famous Food Scientist

The best thing about the future is that it only comes one day at a time.
– Abraham Lincoln

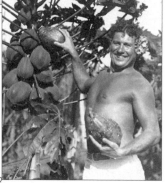

Paul C. Bragg in Tahiti 1920's gathering tropical papaya fruit.

Paul C. Bragg owes his powerful body and superb health to living exclusively on live, vital, healthy, organic rich foods.

Dear Friends – you cannot know how greatly you have impacted my life and some of my friends! We love your Bragg Health Books, teachings and products and are now living healthier, happier lives. Thanks!
– Winnie Brown, Arizona

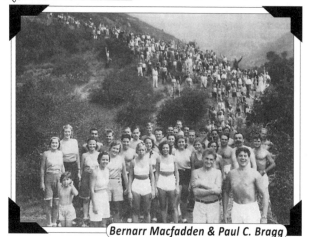

Bernarr Macfadden & Paul C. Bragg

A thousand happy Bragg Health Students enjoy hiking, exercise and fresh air on the trail to Mount Hollywood (above Griffith Observatory) in beautiful California, summer of 1932.

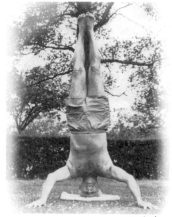

Paul C. Bragg exercising Regent's Park, London.

PAUL & PATRICIA BRAGG

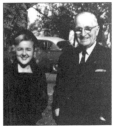

Patricia with 33rd President Harry S. Truman at his home in Independence, Missouri.

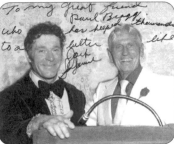

Paul C. Bragg, Creator of Health Food Stores, with his prize student Jack LaLanne, who thanks Bragg for saving his life at 15.

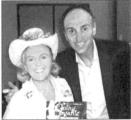

Patrica Bragg with Dr. Jeffrey Smith. He is leader in getting GMO's out of US foods. See GMO video by Jeffrey Smith and narrated by Lisa Oz (Dr. Oz's wife) on web: *GeneticRouletteMovie.com*

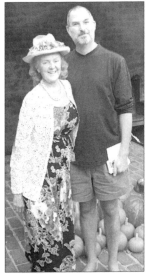

Patricia visiting with Steve Jobs at his home in Palo Alto during the Thanksgiving Holidays.

"I've been reading Bragg Books since high school. I'm thankful for the Bragg Healthy Lifestyle and admire their Health Crusading for a healthier, happier world."
– Steve Jobs, Creator – Apple Computer

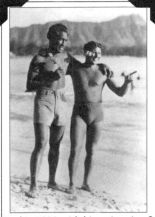

Paul in 1920 with his swimming & surfing friend, Duke Kahanamoku, Waikiki Beach, Diamond Head.

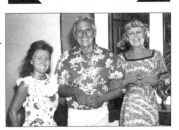

Patricia, Paul C. Bragg and Mrs. Duke (Nadine) Kahanamoku. (Nadine is Patricia's Godmother).

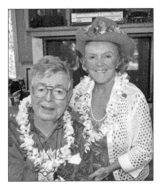

Dr. Earl Bakken with Patricia. He's famous for inventing the first Transistor Pacemaker. His firm Medtronic, developed it and a Resuscitator for fixing ailing hearts that have and are saving thousands of lives. Dr. Bakken lived in Hawaii.

"I cannot remember a time when the Golden Rule ✱ *was not my motto and precept, the torch that guided my footsteps."* – J.C. Penney

✱**The Golden Rule:** Do unto others as you would have them do unto you.

J.C.Penney & Patricia → exercising. They walked often in Palm Springs when he and his wife visited in the winter to enjoy the warm desert sunshine.

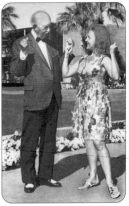

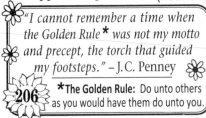

HEALTH CRUSADING TO HOLLYWOOD STARS

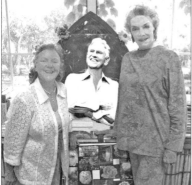

Patricia with friend Actress Jane Russell. Famous Hollywood Star of 40s to 60s.

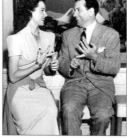

Jane Wyatt learning about health with Paul C. Bragg.

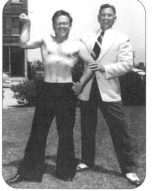

Mickey Rooney with Paul. Rooney was an American film actor and entertainer. He won multiple awards and had one of the longest careers of any actor to age 93!

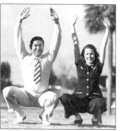

Paul C. Bragg exercising with Actress Helen Parrish.

"Thank you Paul & Patricia Bragg for my simple, easy-to-follow Healthy Lifestyle. You make my days healthy!" – Clint Eastwood, Academy Award Winning Film Producer, Director, Actor and Bragg follower for over 65 years.

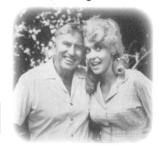

Paul C. Bragg and Donna Douglas, one of Hollywood's most beautiful and talented health advocates. She played the part of "Elly-May" in the *Beverly Hillbillies*, which became one of the longest-running series in television history and was the #1 show in America in its first 2 years.

> Life is a Miracle
> Minute by Minute
> Year by Year!

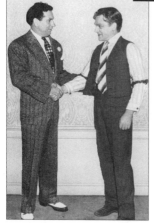

Paul C. Bragg with James Cagney, American film actor. He won major awards for wide variety of roles. The American Film Institute ranked Cagney 8th among the Greatest Male Hollywood Stars of All Time.

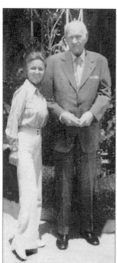

Patricia with Conrad Hilton

← Hotel founder, Conrad Hilton with Patricia Bragg, his Healthy Lifestyle Teacher. *"I wouldn't be alive today if it wasn't for the Braggs and their Bragg Healthy Lifestyle!"* – Conrad Hilton

"Thank you for your website. What a wealth of info to learn about how to live and eat healthy. Many Blessings!" – Michel & Mary, California

207

PHOTO GALLERY

PAUL C. BRAGG, N.D., Ph.D.
PROMOTES HEALTH & FITNESS!

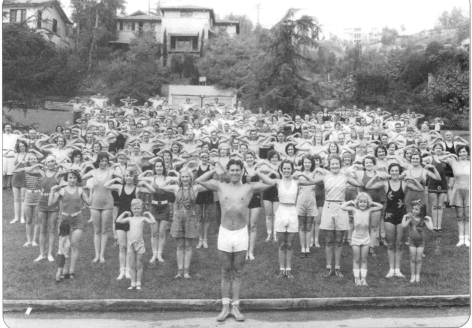

Paul C. Bragg leading an exercise class in Griffith Park, Hollywood, CA – circa 1920s.

Bragg Healthy Lifestyle works Miracles! – Jack LaLanne

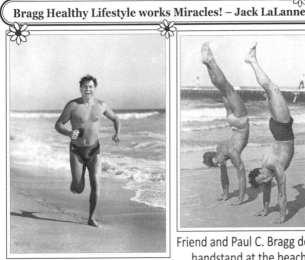

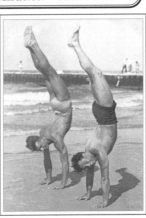

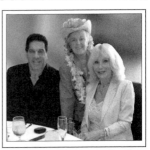

Patricia with Lou and wife Carla at Elaine LaLanne's 90th Birthday Party.

Friend and Paul C. Bragg doing handstand at the beach.

Paul running on Coney Island, New York, where he was a member of the Coney Island Polar Bear Club, known for Cold Water Swimming, 1930s.

TV Hulk Actor Lou Ferrigno gives thanks to Bragg Books. Lou went from puny to become Super Hulk! ➡

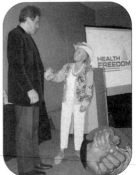

Lou & Patricia in Chicago Health Freedom Expo.

"I lost 102 lbs. with The Bragg Healthy Lifestyle and I have kept it off for over 15 years, staying away from white flour, sugar and other processed foods."
– Dee McCaffrey, Chemist & Diet Counselor, Tempe, AZ

PATRICIA CONTINUING BRAGG HEALTH CRUSADE!

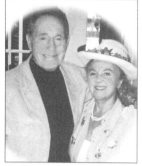

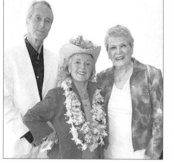

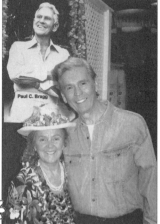

Jack LaLanne with Patricia. Jon & Elaine LaLanne with Patricia.

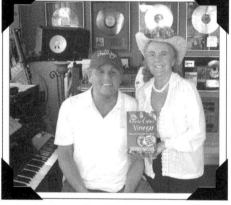

Mother Nature Loves US!

Patricia Bragg with Bill Galt inspired by Bragg Books, he founded Good Earth Restaurants.

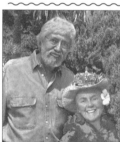

Patricia with Jean-Michel Cousteau Ocean Explorer & Environmentalist. OceanFutures.org

Enjoy a Lifetime of Radiant Health

Patricia in studio with famous Beach Boy Bruce Johnston, Bragg follower over 40 years. He played for her their latest records.

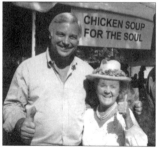

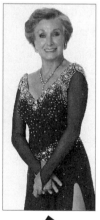

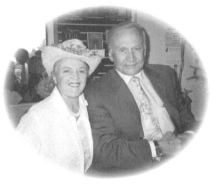

Patricia with Jack Canfield, Bragg follower, Motivational Speaker and Co-Producer of *Chicken Soup For The Soul*.

Patricia with Astronaut Buzz Aldrin, celebrating over 50 years since pilot of Apollo 11 first landed on the moon.

Famous Hollywood Actress Cloris Leachman, ardent health follower who sparkled with health and vitality said, *"The Miracle of Fasting Book is a miracle . . . it cured my asthma, my years of arthritis and many other health problems. I praise Paul and Patricia daily for their Health Crusading!"*

PAUL & PATRICIA BRAGG HEALTH CRUSADING

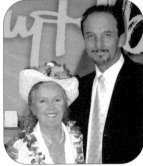

Patricia with Jay Robb.

Paul C. Bragg on the Merv Griffin Show, 1976.

Paul Bragg inspired me many years ago with The Miracle of Fasting Book and his pioneering philosophy on health. His daughter Patricia is a testament to the ageless value of living The Bragg Healthy Lifestyle. – Jay Robb, author of *The Fruit Flush*

During the many years Patricia worked with her father, she was right beside him, assisting him on Bragg Health Crusades worldwide. They were a great team, when you looked at them, you would see only two people headed in the same healthy direction!

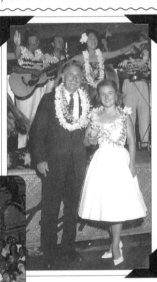

I am a big fan of Paul Bragg. I fast and follow The Bragg Healthy Lifestyle daily. The world and I are blessed with the health teachings of Paul and Patricia Bragg!
– Tony Robbins • TonyRobbins.com

Dream big, think big and enjoy the many miracles.

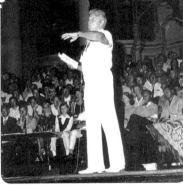

Paul – London Bragg Health Crusade.

Paul & Daughter Patricia, Royal Hawaiian, Honolulu.

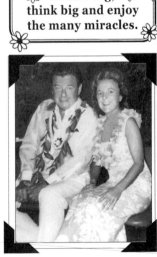

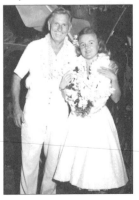

Health Crusaders Paul C. Bragg and daughter Patricia traveled the world spreading health, inspiring millions to renew and revitalize their health.
Bragg Mottos:
3 John 2 and Genesis 6:3

Actor Arthur Godfrey with Patricia, in Honolulu celebrating his 79th birthday.

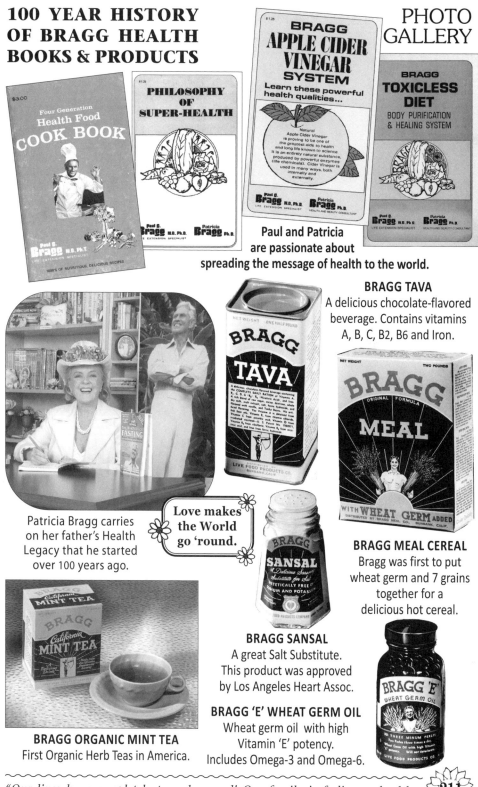

100 YEAR HISTORY OF BRAGG HEALTH BOOKS & PRODUCTS

$3.00

Four Generation
Health Food
COOK BOOK

100'S OF NUTRITIOUS, DELICIOUS RECIPES

Paul C. Bragg N.D. Ph.T.
LIFE EXTENSION SPECIALIST

PHILOSOPHY OF SUPER-HEALTH

Paul C. Bragg N.D. Ph.D.
LIFE EXTENSION SPECIALIST

Patricia Bragg Ph.D.

BRAGG APPLE CIDER VINEGAR SYSTEM
Learn these powerful health qualities...

Natural Apple Cider Vinegar is proving to be one of the greatest aids to health and long life known to science. It is an entirely natural substance, produced by powerful enzymes (life chemicals). Cider Vinegar is used in many ways, both internally and externally.

Paul C. Bragg N.D. Ph.D.
LIFE EXTENSION SPECIALIST
Patricia Bragg Ph.D.
HEALTH AND BEAUTY CONSULTANT

BRAGG TOXICLESS DIET
BODY PURIFICATION & HEALING SYSTEM

Paul C. Bragg N.D. Ph.D.
LIFE EXTENSION SPECIALIST
Patricia Bragg Ph.D.
HEALTH AND BEAUTY CONSULTANT

Paul and Patricia are passionate about spreading the message of health to the world.

Patricia Bragg carries on her father's Health Legacy that he started over 100 years ago.

Love makes the World go 'round.

BRAGG TAVA
A delicious chocolate-flavored beverage. Contains vitamins A, B, C, B2, B6 and Iron.

BRAGG MEAL CEREAL
Bragg was first to put wheat germ and 7 grains together for a delicious hot cereal.

BRAGG ORGANIC MINT TEA
First Organic Herb Teas in America.

BRAGG SANSAL
A great Salt Substitute. This product was approved by Los Angeles Heart Assoc.

BRAGG 'E' WHEAT GERM OIL
Wheat germ oil with high Vitamin 'E' potency. Includes Omega-3 and Omega-6.

"Our lives have completely turned around! Our family is feeling so healthy, we must tell you about it."– Gene & Joan Zollner, parents of 11, Washington

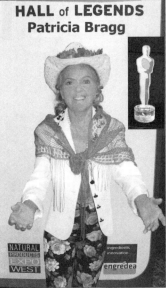

HALL of LEGENDS
Patricia Bragg

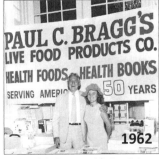

PAUL C. BRAGG'S
LIVE FOOD PRODUCTS CO.
HEALTH FOODS ~ HEALTH BOOKS
SERVING AMERI... 50 YEARS

1962

Paul C. Bragg with Patricia, celebrating over 50 years of Bragg Health Products, Books & Crusading worldwide, spreading Health around the world.

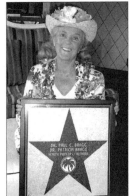

"Palm Spring Walk of Stars" – Patricia with Bragg Star.

Natural Foods Expo in Anaheim with 65,000 attendees from around the world honored Patricia Bragg and her father Paul C. Bragg as treasured Health Food Industry Legends.

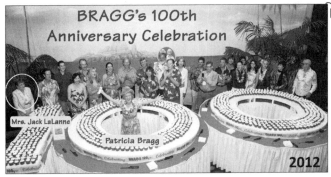

BRAGG's 100th Anniversary Celebration

Mrs. Jack LaLanne

Patricia Bragg

2012

Patricia, Staff & 1,000 Friends celebrated our 100 years of Bragg Healthy Products, Books & Health Crusading! We are proud Pioneers in this Big Health Industry that is helping to keep the world healthier! With Blessings of Health, Peace & Love to You!

Patricia

100 Year Anniversary Party celebrated at the Natural Foods Expo in Anaheim

Bragg Hawaii Exercise Class was founded by Worldwide Health Crusader and Fitness Legend, Dr. Paul C. Bragg. He wanted to create a dynamic, Free Community Exercise Class, and he often taught these classes himself for many years. Patricia Bragg continues her father's health legacy by supporting the Bragg Exercise Class and participates in the class whenever she is in Hawaii.

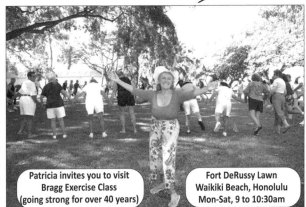

Patricia invites you to visit
Bragg Exercise Class
(going strong for over 40 years)

Fort DeRussy Lawn
Waikiki Beach, Honolulu
Mon-Sat, 9 to 10:30am

"Please make a record of your family history & background. Take pictures – make your own 'Photo Gallery'. Take videos – make movies of your children, spouse, mother and father, family gatherings, etc. These memories are precious & important to save for future generations." – Patricia Bragg

213

The future belongs to those who believe in the beauty of their dreams.
– Eleanor Roosevelt, wife of U.S. President Franklin D. Roosevelt

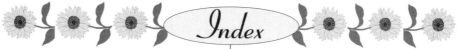

Create the highest, grandest vision for your life, because you become what you believe. – Oprah Winfrey

Dream big, think big, but enjoy the small miracles of everyday life!

Index

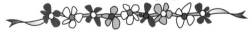

There is no such thing as too many friends, just as there is never too much happiness! – Jean de La Bruyere

---

Wherever there is a human being, there is an opportunity for kindness. – Seneca

---

Self-discipline is your golden key; without it, you cannot be happy.
– Maxwell Maltz, MD – author "Psycho-Cybernetics" and Bragg follower

"You change your life by changing your heart." – Max Lucado

Apple Cider Vinegar - Miracle Health System

BY PAUL C. BRAGG, N.D., PH.D.
and PATRICIA BRAGG

Paul C. Bragg, originator of health stores in America, and world-renowned health crusader Patricia Bragg, introduced America to the life-changing value of Apple Cider Vinegar, with the miracle enzyme known as "the mother." Now a widely popular beverage, this book reveals the legendary health-and life-giving versatility of apple cider vinegar. Following in the footsteps of Hippocrates, who taught the benefits of ACV to his patients in 400 BC, the Braggs teach dozens of reasons to use vinegar, including as a beauty aid, for skin treatments, in recipes, as an antibiotic, anti-septic, hair-revitalizing rinse, headache reliever, and weight reducer. ACV optimizes digestive health and can reduce or eliminate acid reflux. Paul and Patricia Bragg have helped millions heal and restore their vitality and zest for life through their time-tested understanding of natural health. *Apple Cider Vinegar: Miracle Health System* is informative, entertaining, and invaluable for anyone wanting to feel their best.

Bragg Healthy Lifestyle - Vital Living at Any Age

BY PAUL C. BRAGG, N.D., PH.D.
and PATRICIA BRAGG

Learn the simple strategies of radical health and vibrant wellness that The Bragg Healthy Lifestyle has brought to millions! What is an ageless body? For health pioneers Paul C. Bragg and Patricia Bragg, an ageless body sparkles with vitality, immune strength, mental clarity, and digestive ease. The Braggs teach why a toxic-free diet maximizes energy, supports weight loss, and can help heal illness and disease. In the newly revised *Bragg Healthy Lifestyle: Vital Living At Any Age*, the trailblazing father-daughter team who alerted us nearly a century ago to the dangers of sugar and toxic foods, detail every key aspect of creating and maintaining ageless health, including detoxification, stress-release, nutrition, exercise and the importance of taking charge of not only what goes into our bodies, but practices such as fasting, which release the toxins that may unnecessarily accelerate the aging process. "You are what you eat, drink, breathe, think, say and do," is the Bragg motto. From the foods we eat to our outlook, the environments we live in and even in our physical activities, the authors encourage readers to replace toxins with nutrients, flush out poisons and waste efficiently, exercise, breathe deeply and well, and cultivate happiness and harmony in our daily lives.

HEALTH SCIENCE
7127 Hollister Avenue, Suite 25A, Box 249, Santa Barbara, CA 93117
Toll-Free: (833) 408-1122

The Miracle of Fasting - Proven Throughout History

BY PAUL C. BRAGG, N.D., PH.D.
and PATRICIA BRAGG

In this newly revised best-seller, known to millions as the "bible of fasting" health pioneers and researchers Paul C. Bragg and Patricia Bragg teach why this ancient practice is key to health and energy, and critical to longevity and ageless vitality, due to our toxic environment and the stress of our daily lives. They share a detailed, step-by-step approach, accessible and informative for both beginners and experienced fasters. Our bodies must process not only our food and water, but the air we breathe, and whatever chemicals they may contain. Since detoxification and digestion take more energy than even strenuous athletic pursuits, fasting allows the mind and body to rest, renew and regenerate, to come into harmony and balance, and release the effects of stimulating foods like caffeine and sugars. The goal of fasting, say the authors, is to allow for the mind and body to self-heal. This concise, tightly edited *The Miracle of Fasting* is filled with personal stories of Paul C. Bragg's travels around the world, including a fasting journey in India with Mahatma Gandhi.

Healthy Heart - Learn the Facts

BY PAUL C. BRAGG, N.D., PH.D.
and PATRICIA BRAGG

Heart disease claims more American lives than any other illness and is the number one cause of death for women. World-renowned health pioneers Paul C. Bragg and Patricia Bragg teach time-tested, proven strategies for healing and maintaining a healthy heart for a long, active life! In a world filled with technological wizardry and products, the human heart still outperforms them all. That is – if that human heart is kept healthy. That is what the trailblazers Paul C. Bragg and Patricia Bragg have done in this book, sharing simple suggestions for lifestyle changes, nutritional support and exercises that will keep this most miraculous machine, your body, healthy and strong. You will learn how the heart works and how and why coronary disease is preventable and reversible. The authors provide an easy-to-follow blueprint for heart health that includes stress-release techniques, affirming that a positive mental outlook on life is a major element of heart health. The Braggs are legendary in the field of nutrition and health, and this newly revised and edited edition is a foundation of The Bragg Healthy Lifestyle. It is one of the most comprehensive heart health books on the market today.

HEALTH SCIENCE
220 7127 Hollister Avenue, Suite 25A, Box 249, Santa Barbara, CA 93117
Toll-Free: (833) 408-1122

Building Powerful Nerve Force & Positive Energy - Reduce Stress, Worry and Anger

BY PAUL C. BRAGG, N.D., PH.D.
and PATRICIA BRAGG

What is Nerve Force and why should you care about it? According to mental health trailblazers Paul C. Bragg and Patricia Bragg, "Nerve Force" is a type of life energy stored in the nerves, muscles, organs, and brain. The more Nerve Force you have, the quicker you can re-charge it, and the healthier, happier, and more satisfying a life you will lead. If you suffer from burnout, stress, fatigue, anxiety, insomnia or depression, this book is for you! We know that the ability to feel joy and peace is essential to a complete experience of vitality and wellness. Our thoughts, our attitudes, our outlook, and our emotional well-being are all dependent on having a powerful "Nerve Force." Just like any muscle that we can develop and strengthen, we can build our Nerve Force so that we are resilient, relaxed, and calm, even during times of stress. Paul C. Bragg and Patricia Bragg show you how with simple mental exercises and suggestions for specific foods that replenish your Nerve Force, as well as foods that deplete it, in this newly revised edition of *Building Powerful Nerve Force & Positive Energy* the father-daughter team explains to readers the reward of paying attention to the energy that is responsible for not only our physical capabilities and our vital body functions, but our ability to process information and feel centered and grounded, no matter what life throws at us. They teach us that maintaining a healthy Nerve Force, leads to a balanced and fruitful life.

Super Power Breathing - For Optimum Health & Healing

BY PAUL C. BRAGG, N.D., PH.D.
and PATRICIA BRAGG

Do you sometimes find that you are panting instead of breathing? Many of us do! This can cause headaches, anxiety, fatigue, and brain fog. The quality of our breath determines the quality of our life! This book teaches us how to breathe in a way that replenishes the body with the oxygen it so deeply craves. "The more effectively we breathe, the more effectively we live," write the authors, world-renowned health pioneers Paul C. Bragg and Patricia Bragg. "Super Power Breathing can make your life-force stronger, calmer and smarter." The Super Power Breathing program has been followed by Olympic athletes and millions of Bragg followers, and is filled with simple exercises for energizing and rejuvenating your breath, and your whole body. Research shows that we use only one-fourth to one-half of our lung capacity with each breath. This starves our body much like if we are depriving it of food. We are slowly robbing our body of its most vital, invisible nourishment – oxygen. In its newly revised form, the Bragg Super Power Breathing Program will give you all the tools you need to shift from shallow breathing to taking deep, oxygen-filled, life-giving breaths!

Water - The Shocking Truth

BY PAUL C. BRAGG, N.D., PH.D.
and PATRICIA BRAGG

The water you drink can literally make or break your health. The purity of our water is the most critical element in maintaining radical vitality, and healing from illness and disease. In this newly revised edition of *Water: The Shocking Truth*, health crusaders Paul C. Bragg and Patricia Bragg reveal the dangers of tap water, which research shows can be responsible for many ailments, due to the addition of dangerous chemicals such as fluoride and chlorine. In this book, the trailblazing father-daughter team teach the many functions water performs in the body, from regulating the various systems to flushing the body of waste and toxins. But what if the substance we use to cleanse our bodies is itself polluted? With the mandatory fluoridation of water in the municipal water systems, the authors assert that has been the case for decades. Added to the public water supply to prevent tooth decay starting in the 1950s, fluoride has long been known to be a toxin, used in pesticides and rat poisons. Learn what types of water are optimal to drink, how and why to detox your body with nature's most life-giving liquid, and the health-and-life-saving value of installing a water filter in your shower!

Bragg Back & Foot Fitness Program -
Keys to a Pain-Free Back & Strong Healthy Feet

BY PAUL C. BRAGG, N.D., PH.D.
and PATRICIA BRAGG

If you are suffering with back or foot pain, look no further for a comprehensive program that will restore health to the parts of your body that carry you through life! Remember when we were children, and we had the kind of energy and flexibility to play for hours? Agile and active, we could twist, bend, stretch and climb with little effort. However, hours looking at a computer screen, a sedentary lifestyle and poor posture can take their toll. Eventually our backs start to hurt and cramp with every movement, and our feet ache after just a short walk. We start feeling "old." In *Bragg Back & Foot Fitness Program*, the father-daughter team of world-renowned health pioneers, Paul C. Bragg and Patricia Bragg teach how to speed the healing of injuries and develop a strong and flexible back and healthy feet, rejuvenating and re-energizing our bodies in the process. The trailblazing health experts who brought wellness and vitality to millions, including fitness guru Jack LaLanne, outline the keys to a healthy spine, pain-free back and bunion-free feet through nutritional support and clearly illustrated, simple exercises, as well as other tips for posture and massage. Paul and Patricia Bragg reveal the healing properties of herbs, effective ways to practice foot reflexology, how to deal with arthritis, athlete's foot, plantar fasciitis, and foot problems caused by diabetes. By following the authors' Back and Foot Care Program, you can begin to treat your body as Mother Nature intended you to, and creating painless feet, a strong back and a powerful body will begin!

PATRICIA BRAGG
Health Crusader and "Angel of Health and Healing"

Author, Lecturer, Nutritionist, Health & Lifestyle Educator to World Leaders, Hollywood Stars, Singers, Athletes & Millions.

Patricia is a life-long health advocate and activist, admired internationally for her passionate work promoting healthy living. For many years she traveled the world, teaching The Bragg Healthy Lifestyle for physical, spiritual, emotional health and joy. She was invited to give lectures, visited radio shows, was profiled in magazines and appealed to people of all ages, nationalities and walks-of-life. Together with Paul, she co-authored a collection of ten books, with inspiration and techniques for living a long, vital, happy life. Now in her 90s and living on an organic farm in California, Patricia herself is a testament to these teachings and the sparkling symbol of health, perpetual youth and radiant energy.

PAUL C. BRAGG, N.D., Ph.D.
Life Extension Specialist • World Health Crusader
Lecturer and Advisor to Olympic Athletes, Royalty, Stars & Millions.
Originator of Health Food Stores & Founder of Health Movement Worldwide

Paul C. Bragg was at the forefront of the modern health movement, having inspired generations to turn toward wellness. At a young age, Paul turned his own health around by developing an eating, breathing and exercise program to build strength and vitality. From this life-changing experience, he pledged to dedicate the rest of his life to promoting a healthy lifestyle. He opened one of the country's first health food stores, which eventually led to the creation of the Bragg Live Foods company. With a devoted following, Paul traveled giving lectures and sharing his expertise, while serving as an advisor to athletes and movie stars alike. Even Jack LaLanne, the original television fitness guru, credited Paul with having introduced him to the importance of healthy living. In addition to the books Paul wrote with Patricia, they co-hosted television and radio shows and worked together to bring wellness to the world. Paul himself excelled in athletics, loved the ocean and the outdoors, and radiated with health and a warm smile.

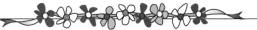

Patricia inspires you to Renew, Rejuvenate and Revitalize your Life with "The Bragg Healthy Lifestyle" Books. Millions have benefitted from these life-changing philosophies with a longer, healthier, happier life!

223

Take Time for 12 Things

1. Take time to **Work** –
    it is the price of success.
2. Take time to **Think** –
    it is the source of power.
3. Take time to **Play** –
    it is the secret of youth.
4. Take time to **Read** –
    it is the foundation of knowledge.
5. Take time to **Worship** –
    it is the highway of reverence and
    washes the dust of earth from our eyes.
6. Take time to **Help and Enjoy Friends** –
    it is the source of happiness.
7. Take time to **Love and Share** –
    it is the one sacrament of life.
8. Take time to **Dream** –
    it hitches the soul to the stars.
9. Take time to **Laugh** –
    it is the singing that helps life's loads.
10. Take time for **Beauty** –
    it is everywhere in nature.
11. Take time for **Health** –
    it is the true wealth and treasure of life.
12. Take time to **Plan** –
    it is the secret of being able to have time
    for the first 11 things.

YOUR BIRTHRIGHT

HEALTH

CULTIVATE IT

Have an
Apple
Healthy Life!

3 John 2

224

*Teach me thy way, LORD, lead me in a straight path,
because of my oppressors. – Psalm 27:11*